D0473983

CANCER SURVIVORSHIP COPING TOOLS

For any woman who has been diagnosed with breast cancer, information is vital. But more importantly, it needs to be good information. Barb's book more than qualifies!

Julie Edstrom, breast cancer survivor, support group facilitator and spiritual director

Mrs. Barbara Tako tells her compelling and poignant real-life journey as she navigates the challenging waters of breast cancer and her life that endures through it all. Well-written. Well-articulated. Easy to read and understand.

Reading this book will be a comfort and encouragement to anyone associated with breast cancer or any other life-threatening disease; whether it be patient, caregiver, family, friends and/or pre-, during, or post-journey.

Throughout the book, Mrs. Tako refers to herself as a "breast cancer survivor." God calls her "more than a conqueror." With the tools and insights in this book, you can be "more than a conqueror" too.

Greg McClain, retired John Deere manager; caregiver for breast and GIST cancer patient for over 12 years

This is a heartfelt and personal account of a patient's walk through breast cancer. Although at times raw, it reveals the triumph of hope and love over trauma and uncertainty. It is full of good advice about education, support groups, coping, and appreciating all the good in life, and will serve as a valuable resource for any newly diagnosed breast cancer (or any cancer) patient.

Dr. Candy Abramson Corey, MD, oncologist and breast cancer survivor

A must-read for those challenged with breast cancer, seeking ideas and inspiration on how to cope with worries accompanying thoughts of surviving today and living tomorrow.

Karmen Mattsen, three-time cancer survivor (Hodgkin's lymphoma, breast, skin)

The author takes us on a reluctant journey. The reader is immersed in the realities and ravages of surgery and chemotherapy. Modern medical therapy offers hope, but always against a background of fear and uncertainty. In the mists of this battleground, the Soul exerts its instinct for freedom. We have choices. Our choices define us, give us clarity, and purpose. Slyly, the author has taken us on a spiritual journey. She exhorts us to make our own journey, and we close the book grateful she has shared hers.

Dr. Kevin Hallman, MD, obstetrician and gynecologist

Sound, practical advice, delivered in a conversation-over-coffee style, for people dealing with any aspect of a breast cancer diagnosis – a book filled with much-needed information.

Anne Johnson, breast cancer survivor since Fall, 1996

Cancer Survivorship Coping Tools – We'll get you through this

Tools for cancer's emotional pain from a melanoma and breast cancer survivor

Cancer Survivorship Coping Tools – We'll get you through this

Tools for cancer's emotional pain from a melanoma and breast cancer survivor

Barbara Tako

AYNI BOOKS

Winchester, UK
Washington, USA

First published by Ayni Books, 2015
Ayni Books is an imprint of John Hunt Publishing Ltd., Laurel House, Station Approach,
Alresford, Hants, SO24 9JH, UK
office1@jhpbooks.net
www.johnhuntpublishing.com
www.ayni-books.com

For distributor details and how to order please visit the 'Ordering' section on our website.

Text copyright: Barbara Tako 2014

ISBN: 978 1 78279 775 3
Library of Congress Control Number: 2014952388

A CIP catalogue record for this book is available from the British Library.

Design: Lee Nash

Printed in the USA by Edwards Brothers Malloy

We operate a distinctive and ethical publishing philosophy in all
areas of our business, from our global network of authors to
production and worldwide distribution.

CONTENTS

Dedicated to

God
Daniel, Emily, and Sarah
All cancer patients — past, present, and future
All cancer caregivers — past, present, and future

Acknowledgements

I am deeply thankful for the support of everyone who helped make this book happen. Above all, I am grateful to a merciful God who was always there with me on my cancer journey.

Special thanks to my friend and publicist Trish Stevens at Ascot Media who supported and encouraged me in every way humanly possible throughout my cancer journey and throughout the writing of this book. Also, many thanks to John Hunt and the rest of the awesome staff at John Hunt Publishing.

Thank you, fellow members of my local breast cancer support group, and all the fellow survivors who helped me. You know who you are! I give extra thanks to Pat Benson for your wonderful insights. I am especially grateful for the support and encouragement of my medical oncology team, my oncology psychotherapist Sandi Tazelaar, my breast cancer support group leader Julie Edstrom, and my very supportive and patient friends Kate Spencer, Anne Johnson, Laura Hutton, Arvilla Cadwell, Jackie and Steve Dimmick, Karmen and Paul Mattsen, Greg McClain, Paulette Henderson, Pam Marta, Jennifer and Jason Lassner, Barb Nevin, Rachel Hanson, Rob and Ike Allickson, and my pastors, Pastor Sue Schoon and Pastor James Woodruff. You all are the best.

Without the love of my family, including David and Anne Seltzer, George and Lucille Tako, Jim Tako, Jan Tako and Nicole Tako, and Tracy Morgan, this book might never have existed. Thank you, dear family!

Last, but not least, I deeply thank my husband Dan and my daughters Emily and Sarah. Your unending love, patience, and support helped me through my cancer journey and inspired me to write this book.

Disclaimer

The author did her best to ensure the accuracy of the quotations, websites, books, and resources mentioned in the text. She assumes no liability, expressed or implied, for any misrepresentations, errors or omissions herein or for any actions taken by readers as a result of the contents of this book.

The author is a writer and a melanoma and breast cancer patient. She assumes no liability for medical or psychiatric advice, expressed or implied herein. For all medical and mental health matters, she refers all readers to their medical and mental health professional providers.

Foreword

It's a journey no one wants to take. A cancer diagnosis propels a person and their family into an unknown world of threshold experiences, intense emotions and a complex system called "health care." It's something I see every day in my work as an oncology psychotherapist. There is initially disbelief and shock that clouds one's rational thinking at a time when the need for critical thinking and decision-making is of utmost importance. This book, *Cancer Survivorship Coping Tools: We'll get you through this*, is a life preserver for those experiencing a cancer diagnosis.

Barbara Tako, a cancer survivor, lends her experiences into a well-thought-out guide to managing a person's medical care, a myriad of emotions, and family/friend/acquaintances' relationships. Her wisdom shines as she leads a person in cutting through the chaos of difficult decisions, and her skill at organizing a framework for sorting through fear, anxiety, sadness and hope is a godsend at such a trying time.

Barbara Tako shares with us her journal entries that people can identify with immediately regarding the rollercoaster effect of the diagnosis, treatment and after-treatment phase of having cancer. She offers hope and an aspect of joy that one feels, upon the diagnosis, has left them for good. Her practical tips and style of writing create an ease in reading that can be translated into regaining emotional resilience with some simplicity.

The research that Tako has done to offer sound advice in addition to her experience is evident. She introduces people to the amazing work done with meditation and breath work that serve to lower one's cortisol, a stress hormone, which increases a sensation of anxiety. Her extensive mention of resources serves to further assist the person facing cancer and their families—it is important to reach outside of one's family for additional support.

This well-written book will be an additional resource that I will freely offer to anyone that is faced with a cancer diagnosis.

Sandi Tazelaar, MSW LICSW
Psychotherapist with a specialty in oncology psychotherapy, 1996 to present

Introduction

We read to know we're not alone.
C.S. Lewis

Dear Reader,

Because this book is in your hands, it most likely means that you or someone you care about has received a cancer diagnosis. As you already know, a cancer diagnosis is a harsh, devastating, life-changing event, regardless of the prognosis and treatment plan. The good news (yes, there *is* good news) is that you are holding in your hands many tools within this book to help get you or your loved one through this journey, starting right now, *and* you are not on this journey alone. I wrote this book because this is the book I wanted to have in my own hands to help me through my own cancer journeys.

This book is intended to be an emotional lifeline. You may sometimes feel very alone and overwhelmed, but you truly are never alone. Whatever you are feeling right now is normal for a very abnormal life event, and there is hope and help for you.

Come on, we will get you *through* this. Even though you may feel swamped, and even though you may feel as though cancer has taken over your entire life forever, 24-7, it won't always feel that way. You won't stay where you are right now, and it is my hope that this book will help you move forward. You will have lots of choices, including some that are suggested in this book. Choices can be positive and give you back some control. If you have a chance, please write or e-mail and let me know how your journey is going.

Section I

Explanations and Tools for Coping with Your Diagnosis

You are braver than you believe, stronger than you seem, and smarter than you think.
Winnie the Pooh

Who I Am and Who I Am Not

My name is Barbara and I am a breast cancer and melanoma cancer survivor. May 6, 2010 was my personal 9/11. I was 46 years old at the time of my first cancer diagnosis—my breast cancer diagnosis. To date, I have made it through two surgeries, chemotherapy, radiation, some bouts with lymphedema, and several other complications, and then, several years out, a melanoma that wasn't in the area where I had radiation. My story is unique, just as yours is.

We are each unique on this journey

We each have a different type, grade, stage, and prognosis for our cancer. We come into cancer at different ages and with different health situations. Our emotional make-ups, our social networks, our family situations, our stages of life, our belief systems, and our faiths are all different. Yet, we have all heard the words "You have cancer." We have all experienced the emotional pain and life-changing upheaval from hearing that. Regardless of our cancer type, we share some common threads as we work to weave our cancer diagnosis into the fabric of our lives, get through it, and move onward. Try not to compare yourself to others. Whatever you may be feeling right now is normal. Truly, it is okay to feel what you are feeling. This is your journey and you are allowed to think what you think, feel what you are feeling, and, most importantly, to simply be yourself. We will get you through this.

As for me, I am not an expert. I am not a medical professional or a counseling professional. I am not even a "good" patient. Maybe it is *because* I am not a good patient that this book exists. I struggled a lot with my breast cancer diagnosis. I was very upset, anxious, and afraid. I felt isolated, inexperienced, and forever changed. This book exists because of the many overwhelming feelings that I experienced. The devastating fear, loneliness, intense relentless anxiety, and grief led me to seek out a lot of information and resources to get myself through this, and I did not do it alone.

Getting to a better place took time and dead ends, and much patience from family, friends, and professionals, but I learned a lot. I want to share what I learned to help you. I would like my long, gradual learning curve to emotional cancer survivorship to be your shorter, quicker one. Please pick and choose. You will find things here that will help you get through this. Above all, don't give up. We *will* get you through this. You are not alone (even at 2:00 a.m. when you are upset and can't sleep). There are tools here to help you. Pick and choose what works for you and, please, disregard the rest.

Who I Was

Before cancer, I was a Christian* wife, mother of two, motivational clutter-clearing and home-organizing speaker, and published author. Life was pretty good (life is pretty good now, too, just different). I didn't want to be a breast cancer survivor. Who does? I didn't like the color pink (and I still don't), and I wanted nothing to do with cancer at all. Who would? I liked living with my head in the sand and operating under the commonly shared illusion that life would just chug merrily along forever, or that if things should happen to take a bad turn, I would somehow be magically ready for those events if/when they finally came. Hah.

*A note about my Christian faith. My faith is part of my belief system. Expressions pertaining to my faith in this book are not intended to sound preachy or in any way push you to substitute your belief system for mine. I try to be honest here about my personal faith, *and* I recognize that everyone has different images of God, so I trust you to reference your own source when you come across my references in this book. If the faith-based comments in this book make you uncomfortable, I encourage you to fast-forward past them for other ideas and suggestions here that may be helpful to you.

Why This Book

After my cancer diagnosis, through treatment and beyond, I wanted to *feel* better. I understood I had cancer and it needed to be treated. Those were the physical aspects of this disease. I understood the possibility of cancer returning was a new worry I would have for the rest of my life. I didn't understand, with all the medical information and help out there, why there wasn't something that could help me help myself to better manage the worry and to *feel* better. I began to work on compiling the thoughts, information, experiences and resources that helped me deal with the sometimes overwhelming feelings. As I did this, I began to wish someone could just put a book in my hands that would help me reduce the emotional pain I was feeling. The need and desire for that book is why this book exists. I wrote the book I wished someone had handed to me.

The cancer journey is a marathon instead of a sprint.

Personally, I do better at sprints than marathons, but hey, cancer didn't ask me what my preference is! Even if you are a former sprinter, you can move yourself forward in this process. You can learn marathon skills. You are not stuck even if you feel stuck or swamped by your diagnosis. Time and working through your experience will move you along. It does get better.

There is more good news! We can expand the tools in your emotional backpack *now*. Right now. No waiting. Read on and move yourself forward. First, we can vent and clarify the loss, and then we can assemble our weapons to fight back.

This book is divided into three sections: Diagnosis, Active Treatment, and After Treatment. Throughout, I share excerpts from my breast cancer and melanoma cancer journaling and include tools to help at each part of the process. The cancer experience isn't a steady linear process. There are spikes and dips, and sometimes circular events or circular thinking (oh, yeah). You may find a tool under Diagnosis that is actually more helpful to you After Treatment. You may choose to skip to the section that fits best where you are right now, or you may choose to read the book in the order it is written.

Whatever approach you use, be patient, kind and gentle with yourself. If something you read doesn't fit for you, it is my fault — not yours. Simply disregard it. If it is better to put this book down or step away for a while, that may be the best thing for you at the moment. Follow your own instincts. Some cancer patients seek help to get through the treatment experience. Others put blinders on, get through treatment, and then may emotionally collapse after the finish line and choose to sort it out afterwards. There is no single right way to deal with this tough stuff!

Above all, remember you are not alone and we will get you through this, starting right now.

What Finding Out You Have Cancer Might Feel Like

By having the courage to be yourself, you put something wonderful in the world that was not there before.
Edwin Elliot

Here is what my diagnosis felt like. This is an excerpt from my journal—your experience will feel different but you may relate to parts of this:

Sunday, June 20
My oncology therapist suggested that I hadn't written in my journal (other than a few factual entries in the last month about my breast cancer) because the breast cancer diagnosis was *too big*. Here goes.

Yes, it is too big. I feel steamrolled, overwhelmed, shifted to a different train track where the ride is much faster, wilder, and bumpier, and I am lost. I also realize I am just getting started. My life has changed completely forever. I have switched train tracks. I *hate* that this fear and worry will hang over me for the rest of my life—even my gynecologist said the shadow of this would be there for the rest of my life. He also said this will take its pound of flesh, and yes, it certainly has.

I was diagnosed on May 6, 2010 with invasive ductal carcinoma (IDC) in the right breast. It was caught on a routine mammogram. My oncotype score had a 10-year recurrence percentage in the high intermediate range. That meant the cancer had a pretty high chance of coming back! To improve the odds for keeping cancer away, it meant that for me, chemotherapy would be part of my treatment.

With chemo, I have a pretty good prognosis. Except, right now, I am not feeling very lucky—getting breast cancer wasn't lucky, and being one of the ones who would also have chemo (instead of radiation only, which, before the oncotype results,

5

was the plan), *wasn't* lucky. I am upset and I am getting a little out of order.

I got the first call, the notification that I had breast cancer, from my doctor while I was sitting in my car at the gas station I sometimes stop at on Thursday mornings. It was my fault. I had rolled my home phone to my cell phone "just in case" to get his call. It's like 9/11 except this one is only for me. It is my personal 9/11. It is a date and location I will always remember. In an instant, I was separated and isolated from all the people around me going through their normal daily life business. I went on to my next appointment of the day and cried the whole time. I cried a lot since then too.

Everyone's story is a little different. Our ages, lifestyle, views, spirituality, relationships, and specific types of cancer are each unique. Everyone's choices, reactions and experiences with cancer or breast cancer are different too. This is just mine:

For the record, I had anxiety issues *before* this whole thing started (heavy sigh). Of course...

I thought I got through the initial research, finding a good surgeon, and having a lumpectomy pretty well. I was blessed to connect with a friend through my church who was going through a similar cancer diagnosis. I was blessed it was caught early on a mammogram. I even had "good days" where I could get my mind off it for a while with gardening or exercise, *then* I found out I would be going through chemotherapy. I was at home when the call came. I found myself down on the floor crying. I didn't know much about chemo, but I knew it meant hair loss, more separation from those around me, a much longer active treatment period and more unhappy side effects too.

I find a great breast cancer support group locally. I am blessed to have a kind, loving, supportive husband who is trying his absolute best to help me through this. I am happiest when I am asleep (I think that is kind of sad, but I heard another breast cancer survivor mention that too at the support group meeting this week).

My lumpectomy was on May 19. It went well. I went home numb rather than in pain. I threw away the prescription painkillers. I was not brave. It was because narcotics make me severely nauseated—I didn't want to be wrenching around to throw up with fresh incisions in my torso. I got through the first few days of surgery with ice and ibuprofen. It worked. My scars look like wide red scratches. I have one about 2½ inches across the top of my right breast and one about half that size under the right arm where the surgeon removed two lymph nodes.

Now I have started chemotherapy (June 14) the day before I turn 47. Happy Birthday. The sometimes "good days" appear to be gone. Anxiety, huge mood swings, pain and fatigue. Long term. This isn't going well. Can't go over it. Can't go under it. Can't go around it. Must go through it. No choice. I really *hate* that. I hate that cancer and its treatment will take a terrible toll on my body. I really, really hate that it feels like it will be a shadow that hangs over my head for the rest of my life. I hate being weak and tearful and sad and sore and different—forever different.

Sometimes I don't understand why people don't run away from me. I would run away from this if I could. To clarify, I wouldn't run from a friend, but I would run from my disease if I could.

I hate that I am a glass-is-half-empty sort of person and that everyone says that to beat it, it really helps to have a positive attitude. I feel like I am going to turn inside out and explode. It isn't that I am not trying. I am seeing a therapist, taking anti-anxiety medications, exercising when I can, staying hydrated, trying to eat well, and managing the medications to keep the chemo side effects manageable. I am trying the guided imagery and positive affirmation tapes too.

There are tears when the days get too long and overwhelming. I just hurt. Pain wakes me up to be with *it* in the middle of the night. My head. My back. My hips. Now my knees hurt too. I love my husband and daughters. I love my family and friends. I want to fight this. I want to fight this for me and for all the people who care about me. I just feel sore, battered, beat-up, and like I am only at the start of what is going to be a long journey. I can't see as far as tomorrow at this point. I miss Sarah, my youngest daughter—she just left for music camp for two weeks. I miss my husband Dan (he drove her with his brother to help). Emily, my eldest daughter, stayed with me and did her best to try to help me.

I think the pain is the hardest. It is a reaction to the white-count-boosting Neulasta shot: I woke up at 3:00 a.m. this morning crying from lower back pain that lasted until about 6:00 p.m. Sunday night. The on-call doctor, on the second phone call, prescribed something that started to help after several hours. Pain doesn't let you forget. Not for a minute...

Do we have some feelings in common? That is more than enough about me for now. I really want you to understand you are not alone. The American Institute for Cancer Research says, "The moment you are diagnosed with cancer, you join approximately fourteen million other survivors in the US alone."

Let's work on getting you through your story. Yes, you will get *through* this. First, take a deep breath and consider what just happened to you. You know it is huge and life-changing, yet it is different for each of us in terms of diagnosis, prognosis, life stage, past experience, emotional response, treatment plan, and time frame to name just a few aspects. Even with differences, there are some common themes.

There can be feelings of pain, fear, anger, isolation, loneliness, grief and defenselessness. That is a string of pretty negative adjectives, and they are very real. I would also add words that don't readily come to mind. For me, cancer felt relentless, continuous, all-encompassing and overpowering. I felt swamped by it. It took over everything else. It was exhausting.

My friend Trish, when describing her own cancer scare, put it this way:

> Absolutely no one can ever understand the attack on your mind, your spirit and what it mentally does to you—until they have been told they have cancer. Your world becomes turned upside down. Fear takes over your whole being. Thoughts take over your entire mind. Things you've never thought of in your life overwhelm you suddenly. Coping with everything and anything becomes almost impossible. Shock stays within you and you just walk around, in tears, tired all of the time, even in pain, and in fear... while everyone else just cannot relate and has no clue of the depth of what you are going through. Sometimes it seems as if they are completely blind to what you are going through, and that hurts, but it's because they cannot feel it as you do. Every symptom you feel makes you want to pick up a medical book and research to see if something else is now going wrong in your body. We know we have to 'think' positively, but our fears are too strong and we don't know 'how' to think positively.

Do you feel derailed and defenseless from your diagnosis? Are the usual tools you have used in the past for attitude adjustment or calming yourself not working so well *this* time? If so, it is understandable given the magnitude of what has happened to you. *Many breast cancer survivors I have spoken with say that the emotional aspects of the diagnosis were more difficult than the physical difficulties from treatment.* That is pretty compelling considering the physical difficulties and pain that go with surgeries, chemotherapy, and radiation.

Maybe you feel terribly alone and you would like someone to just be there with you, to simply sit next to you and be there emotionally. Maybe you want help to go forward in this frightening new emotional terrain. You are not alone. Repeat. You are not alone. Keep reading and you will see that this is true. Keep breathing. Keep believing. Keep moving forward. Keep breathing. You can learn the tools of cancer survivorship.

What You Might Need or Want Right Now

Be wise in the use of time. The question in life is not how much time do we have. The question is what shall we do with it.
Anna Robertson Brown, author

Think about what you need and begin by writing it down. Here is a list from my journal as I experienced breast cancer treatment. Hopefully checking out the list below and thinking about your wants will continue the process of moving you forward.

What I would want, as a cancer patient, looking back (hindsight, of course, is 20-20)

1. To be connected with people. (I felt isolated by my diagnosis.)
2. To be distracted. (I would have given anything for a few minutes not thinking about cancer.)
3. To celebrate and focus on the positives, any positive, more. (Like the great people I met and the things I learned about myself.)

4. To be heard. (It was nice when someone would really listen and help me process the cancer experience.)

5. To *know*, without self-blaming, that the mood swings and emotions, especially the fear, are a normal part of this unfortunate process. (This was *huge* for me.)

6. To not beat myself up for anything I felt or thought or did during this journey—especially during treatment. (No self-beating. This journey is hard enough as it is.)

7. To somehow pamper myself more in this treatment period and afterward while recovering from treatment. (My friend Laura put it best by always encouraging me to be gentle with myself—to treat myself the same way I would want to encourage a friend in the same situation.)

8. To engage my senses more, especially to pet my dogs and hug my family more, and keep my hands busy with a craft, any craft or puzzle or sorting process, something. (Focusing on external senses instead of worrisome cancer thoughts.)

9. To stay in the moment more and to stop my worried thoughts from racing ahead to the future thinking about dire outcomes. (Stay in the present. Don't jump to dire conclusions. You are alive right now.)

The Loss

What does finding out you have cancer feel like? Here is another journal entry. It was homework assigned to me by my oncology therapist (more about that later). I am including it here because I think it was good homework, important homework, for you to consider doing too.

Journal Tool

Before we can get through something, I think it helps if we take the time to define it. Please consider keeping your own journal and taking the time, in writing, to vent, define, and process your own loss and experiences. Let them out. Help all those thoughts and feelings get out of spinning around in your head. Write them down. Journal entries can be as long or short as you need them to be. You can journal several times in a day or only once a week. There is no one right way to journal. Be honest in your journal. Please try it. Here is my journal entry and therapy homework:

November 4

Observation: I don't like this homework from my therapist. What if it is unending, all the realizations and nuances? Isn't even one paragraph of life with cancer bad enough?

The loss from my breast cancer diagnosis and journey changes my life in so many ways forever. It is hard to write about this loss because it feels so enormous and comprehensive, even with a very good prognosis and even emerging from this with my two original breasts, a slimmer body, and hair that now has some curl. The breast cancer journey isn't one loss. It is many.

There is a loss of innocence about the bad things that can happen to someone and the depth and variety of ways those losses can hurt. When I hear and read about and see other people's trouble, cancer or not, I hurt in a deeper way every time. I feel sad about the state of the world we live in and the suffering we all experience in so many ways.

Personally, I am sad that I have permanently lost who I was and how I felt as a person before the breast cancer diagnosis. I do believe in and look forward to a "new normal," but it won't be the same, and I mourn that and rage against it a lot.

There is a deep sadness in me because the shadow of this journey will hang over me for the rest of my life. I have been told it gets better over time and I believe that, or I might not have made it this far, except for my faith and wonderful family and caring friends, but I am sad it will never go away. I believe I can beat breast cancer. I believe I have a very good chance to beat it.

I also know, as a competitive person, that I can't "win" this life event that happened to me. I can't make it go away, now or ever. As hard as I try to do all the right things (prayer, diet, exercise, information, support from family, friends, and professionals...) I can't undo what happened to me. It isn't my decision as to whether or not the breast cancer comes back for me. Having had breast cancer will be part of me for the rest of my life. That hurts and it makes me very, very sad and angry. I can't get my "A." I want to undo all of this. I can't. I struggle to accept that.

I will always feel like a middle-aged person that was thrust forward in time to experience worries that many people don't face until later in life. I can't undo what I have experienced, heard, felt, and seen. I have lost some part of my middle age that I don't think I can entirely get back. It is sad but it also is a gift. I know, at a gut level at age 47, how mortal I am and how random and unfair the universe can be. What will I do with that knowledge? How can I use it for good? That is the challenge.

With a breast cancer diagnosis, there are worries that will never go away. There are things I can't fix and make right. I will always see the scar on my chest and have lymphedema worries for the rest of my life. I will always have to watch my body more carefully for the rest of my life. (Also, the doctors will watch me more carefully too.)

Physically, will I ever feel the same again? If so, I think it will take a long time. The chemo, radiation, surgeries, medications and stress have each taken their toll on my body, my face, my thoughts and my emotions. Move forward, yes.

Completely recover? I just don't know, and I mourn that.

I will always need to be very diligent about scheduling my physicals and mammograms. I will always worry more now for the rest of my life every time I have a mammogram, physical, x-ray, blood work, or any other health check.

I will always worry that because my nature has been glass-is-half-empty that, in spite of all my efforts to do the "right" things, I am hurting my good prognosis (though even the American Cancer Society website says this isn't a factor). *I have lost the ability to not worry about cancer coming back as a recurrence or metastasis, and the pain and suffering, and maybe even death that could come with it.* There it is in one sentence.

In more details, there will always be the worry of future health issues that can happen from the chemo, radiation, long-term medication, and surgeries. I will always notice and react more when the word "cancer" comes up in conversation, on the radio, on television, or on the Internet. I feel like I will always have more fear in my life than I had before this. Always. Always. Always. These things won't go away no matter how much I want them to go away.

Another loss is the loss of time. I was diagnosed on May 6, 2010. I was told at my clinic that I won't feel like myself or "get my body back" until *maybe* March of 2011. [January 16, 2011: That was before C-diff and surgery to remove my ovaries and uterus.] I feel like I have lost five months of my life already in many ways, and it sounds like I will lose more.

I am sad at the time lost helping my daughters, Emily and Sarah, and being there for Dan, my husband, who has been generous, patient, wonderful, supportive, and kind through this entire journey. He has given me so much. How can I tell and show him how much I love him? I know marriage isn't a place to keep score, but I don't know how to repay him or my daughters. I love them so much.

I have lost things I can't change as I learned through this

journey. I think about the emotional temper tantrums and acting out that my daughters witnessed. Yes, I have broken many family-of-origin patterns, but some things did happen. I can't undo those for my daughters or make them go away. Some of my behavior was not a good example or model for them. Those are losses I can't take back. I will be sorry about them for the rest of my life.

There is also the loss of some of my daughters' innocence when we tell them about the hereditary component to this disease and that they will need mammograms and closer health monitoring at 36 years old rather than the usual age. I will also tell them about the importance of diet and exercise as prevention. My breast cancer has caused this for them. It can't be undone. Of course, I hope there is a cure or better treatments or that this will be a nonissue for both of them in their lives. Regardless, some of their innocence will be lost.

I am sad about the time I have lost and am losing enjoying life with my family and my friends. I can't get that time back. Will I enjoy life again? I think I am ungrateful for my good prognosis, yet even without self-beating for feeling this way, it is how I feel.

I have lost some of the precious time and energy to market my first book, my sort-of-third baby, and my legacy to this world in some ways, because of the timing of the breast cancer. I mourn that I can't do more right now to "save my baby" (a book gets its best marketing shot when it is new, that is, less than one year old) because of my distress and fatigue.

My oncology therapist says *I have lost certainty*. That sums it up best. I will live the rest of my life with uncertainty. As a person who likes the illusion of control, I am not happy with that.

Does that sound depressing? I was pretty depressed when I wrote it. The funny thing is that now, each time I go back and read it, I feel *stronger*. I feel like I have moved past a lot of it. I can't make it go away, but I can work through it and move forward and you can too!

In addition to the journal entry/homework assignment above, I also kept a running list about what was upsetting me. It felt good to get each of these thoughts out of my head (or *less* in my head) by putting them down on paper. Journaling these ideas can be extremely helpful. You can try this too. Here is the list from my journal:

Things that bother me about having and recovering from breast cancer

1. Conflicting information regarding breast cancer, treatment, and nutrition from reading and from healthcare professionals themselves. I can make myself crazy (okay, crazier) by reading too much.

2. Emotional downs (chemo-created, hormonally related, surgically created, self-inflicted/ingrained, long-term worry).

3. Anxiety—fear of recurrence, fear of metastasizing, fear of death, fear of somehow "not doing treatment right."

4. Cancer thoughts, fears, and worries taking over so much of my mind so constantly, especially in the early months of this journey.

5. Driving my friends and family away—either when I am hurting if I push people away or when I just figure they are sick of my one-topic conversation, or I figure that they are tired of my tears—huh, really not my decision to make, is it?

6. Having cancer worries and fears hanging over my head for the rest of my life.

7. Worrying about possible cancer or other physical damage from the chemo, radiation, and follow-up drugs.

8. Hair loss. Yes, hair grows back, but this issue is still *huge*, and visible, and therefore public.
9. Fatigue.
10. Pain. Pain from drugs. Pain from surgeries. Worries about causes of pain.
11. Feeling overwhelmed by what used to be just considered normal life.
12. Hot flashes—hot and sweaty, cold and clammy with no middle "normal" temperature for me.
13. Lack of sleep.
14. Breast scar.
15. Uncertainty. "Loss of certainty" (my oncology therapist said this most simply). Living with uncertainty on a gut level and a mental level for the rest of my life.

There are some things I love about the above list that I think are worth mentioning here. Yes, I said "love." I *love* that I could write these awful things down. Writing them down did help get them onto paper and out of my head! It was a huge relief to articulate each thought in my journal and let it go (at least somewhat).

I *love* that I can read these items and learn from them and take a little bit of their power away each time I read my list. I especially love that it is a *finite* list. If you had asked me to guess how long this list would be early in my journey, I would have said it would be over one hundred items long. Not true. I love that. Your list will be limited too. Did you hear that? I said *limited*.

The Shock of Diagnosis

Recognize you are at the beginning. This is Ground Zero. You have heard the words "You have cancer."

Allow yourself to feel what you feel. Give yourself permission to feel whatever you are feeling. This is *major*. In all honesty, there may be other points on this journey where you feel this bad or this strongly but at this point, those feelings are also combined with the shock and the newness of what has just happened to you.

If you can, find someone close to be with you as you experience the shock of the initial awareness of the loss. It could be a family member or a friend who is good at giving hugs.

This may also be a good time to draw strength from your faith. It might be helpful to contact your religious leader. My faith background is Christian, but it is not my intent to push my religious beliefs onto you. We all have different faith/spirituality stories and backgrounds, and I apologize in advance if any of my thoughts or references in this book are in any way pushy or offensive. The thoughts I share are only my own very personal and individual experience.

You could get in contact with someone who is further on the path of a cancer journey similar to your own. Their perspective could be very helpful for you. Some hospitals and clinics now have "cancer buddy" programs where you can be matched with someone with a similar diagnosis who is a little further out on their cancer journey. Sometimes a friend of a friend knows someone who has been through a diagnosis like yours. A personal contact like this can help with feelings of isolation and the loneliness of the diagnosis.

Allow yourself room to cry and grieve. Try to find a place that you feel safe. Seek and hang on to whatever you find to be comforting at this point. It might be a glass of wine or a television show or movie. It might be a soft blanket and a comfortable place on the couch. Maybe it is a safe nest in your bed. Figure out where you feel the most comforted and protected right now *and go there*.

Maybe you are wondering how you got cancer? Perhaps you

are wondering what you did wrong? Are you thinking about nature versus nurture and wondering if one or the other or both contributed to your cancer? That is normal now too. Again, I say be gentle with yourself.

Maybe you are worrying about changes to your body (surgeries) or hair loss from possible upcoming chemotherapy. These very real possibilities can loom very large in your mind. It is hard for those thoughts not to be there with a breast cancer diagnosis because of all the attention our society pays to women's hair and breasts. Try not to look too far down the road yet. There is some great support out there to help deal with these events if necessary—and I will say that my wig tended to look nicer than my hair ever did and that many survivors I have spoken to were extremely pleased with the skill of their surgeons. It is normal to be worried about these things, but do not despair.

As you progress through those first, shocking, intense waves of feelings, try to sort out and begin building your emotional toolbag from the chapters that follow. It may be redundant to mention some of the things in the next chapters, but perhaps if they are mentioned, it may raise your awareness and they can be better utilized to help you.

The Active Cancer Treatment Period Doesn't Go On Endlessly

When I received my cancer diagnosis, it felt like my life had changed forever. The treatment window for most of us though, including me, is limited. A lot of the most difficult stuff won't go on forever. I remember a fellow survivor at a breast cancer support group meeting commenting that when she was diagnosed, someone pointed out that 12–18 months out, she would be done with the worst parts of the active cancer treatment process and be able to be back to her usual life. That made it feel more doable!

The active treatment window is finite. In many ways, you will get your life (and hair) back after active cancer treatment. I won't say that there aren't some scary things to get through or that everyone has a pretty good prognosis, but try to keep this perspective. You can get through this!

The timeline can vary depending on the diagnosis and treatments, but it is the perspective here that is worth remembering. This upsetting life-changing event that may include surgeries, chemo, and radiation won't, for most of us, be a never-ending process. You will get through those things and come out on the other side of active cancer treatment as a wiser and stronger person. Hang in there.

Safe Place Tool

Help yourself by finding a safe place in your home—a cozy spot where you feel safest. It could be your bed, the end of the couch, or a special chair. Add your most tactile and soothing blanket. When you feel upset, go there. Burrow in! Take a break! You are trying to wrap your head and your emotions around this frightening diagnosis. Go to your safe place and try to redirect your thoughts for a while. Focus on the comfort of being in a safe place. When you are in your safe place, you aren't having a surgery, you aren't having chemotherapy, and you aren't in a doctor's office. You are safe.

Friends and Family

You may be surprised here, or not. Many of your friends and family may rally around you when they learn what has happened. Or you may be in a situation where you don't have a lot of friends or family near you. There also may be family members or friends who just can't go there—who just can't deal with you with cancer. If some react that way to you, please realize their reaction is not about you. It is about them. Hopefully, others may step up to support you or you may find more help from some of the other tools mentioned in this book. It is important to reach out to those who can help you. If you can't reach out, consider seeing a mental health professional to explore why you aren't able to reach out. Connecting for people support can be very helpful.

If friends or family are there for you, take comfort in their love and support when it is offered. In addition to the people you expect to be there, you may find some of your more distant friends may step up to the plate and take an active and supportive role for you. You may even find yourself surprised by kindness from strangers—perhaps those who have been there themselves or have had loved ones touched by cancer.

If you do not have a spouse, close friends, or nearby family, you still are not alone. Reach out and connect with others who have been through, or are currently on the cancer journey. Also, a little secret, whether we have a lot of external support or only a little, we all feel shocked, frightened and alone with our cancer.

I hope you have at least one person in your life who can just be there with you in the grief and shock of what has happened to you, one person who can sit and cry and be sad and be angry and be hurt with you. It doesn't always require conversation or problem-solving at this point. Sometimes it is nice to have someone to be there with you as you sit in the bottom of the hole you suddenly feel you have accidentally fallen into.

You may also find some friends and family who don't handle

your diagnosis well. From my experience, I say try to just leave them be. You can't change other people, and you already have more than enough to manage. Let it go, and focus on the support you *are* receiving from others.

Things will be different. This is a new journey for you and for the people around you. Your treatment may impact your relationships, including your sex life. Your priorities and focus may change. Your body may change too. What you seek in your relationships with others may be different.

On a related note, one dear friend brought up an important point. She said that at some point in my cancer journey, she and/or others who care deeply for me may hurt me, not on purpose, but accidentally by something they say or don't say, or do or don't do. She was right. At one point, this dear friend herself said something that didn't sit right with me. I don't really think it was anybody's "fault." Our friendship was close and I remembered her advice so that I could mention it to her shortly after it happened. We dealt with it and moved on. What I would like to suggest to you is that a close friend or family member isn't psychic and isn't perfect. Don't instantly mentally relegate them into the mental category of "someone I can't share this with" because of one or two things that don't work for you. Recognize that they love you and they are trying their best, whatever that looks like at the moment.

If you can talk to them about it, talk. If you can just let it go, do so. You and they are there for the duration. In talking about marriage, my grandfather used to say, "It doesn't matter if you lose the battle. What matters is winning the war." Cancer is the same kind of thing. It is a marathon, not a sprint.

A little bit down the road... make lists

After the shock and initial pain, you will be finding yourself thinking of a million questions and wanting to make a treatment plan to deal with the cancer.

It is important to have good resources and information for the difficult decisions you will be making about your treatment.

It is a good time to start making lists of questions. In fact, make written lists of anything going on in your head. It is good to get those thoughts and questions out of spinning around in your head and down on paper instead.

Again, you may find it helpful to talk to someone who has been through this before. You can seek out local cancer support groups or ask for a phone call from a survivor (try the American Cancer Society).

Medical Team

This is the time when you put together your medical team. That is, you will be assembling a team of doctors for yourself—perhaps a surgeon, medical oncologist and radiation oncologist. To create this team—ask, ask, ask everyone around you for their doctor experiences and what doctors their friends with cancer used. Call the American Cancer Society with any questions too. ACS won't suggest specific doctors, but they will help you ask good questions.

Consider meeting more than one doctor in each specialty you need. Get second opinions from surgeons, medical oncologists, and radiation oncologists. Go to appointments with written lists of questions. Ask. Ask. Ask.

It is critical for your emotional health to create a team of doctors that you trust with your care, and then, trust them! A belief in your medical team will be a strong pillar to help get you through this cancer process. It is empowering and positive to have a medical team and a plan as you move forward.

Suggestion: As you explore doctors, find out how many cases like yours that the doctors you are considering have treated. I am not a doctor or qualified to give medical advice. I just personally think that amount of experience counts for something.

Another suggestion: Create two folders: one for the medical information you will be compiling, including pathology reports, blood tests, doctor information, and one folder of items for taking care of you—references, suggestions for support groups, coupons for pedicures or massages...

A Word about Internet Usage

Is the Internet a great resource for cancer patients or a frightening one? The Internet can be a mixed bag for a cancer patient. On the one hand, there is this tremendous source of information and contact with fellow cancer patients right at your fingertips. On the other hand, there may be inaccurate, incomplete or contradictory information out there as well.

Discussion boards can be a mixed blessing. It can be comforting and helpful to connect with other cancer patients around the country or around the world, but it can sometimes become confusing and even frightening. Each person's experience and circumstances are unique. Sometimes a discussion or posting can raise more questions and worries than it can answer. Often someone posts because they are having concerns, as people tend not to post when things are going well. It is human nature to do this but it means the information out there can be worrisome. However, just because something happened to the person in the post doesn't mean it will happen to you. Whenever you find a piece of information on the Internet, consider the credibility of the source and recognize that you don't know the whole medical story of the person who posted it.

A fellow patient may be a different age or have a different

medical history, family history, prognosis, or treatment plan than you do. Sometimes you might think you are comparing apples to apples when you may not be doing that at all. Is what you find backed up by credible research? What does your own team of doctors have to say?

Approach the Internet carefully.

Create a medical team for yourself that you trust
I will say it again. I can't overemphasize the importance of building a medical team and game plan to fight the cancer that you are comfortable with and that you believe is the best for you. It can be frustrating that, at the very moment you want to crawl under a rock, you need to reach out, educate yourself, and make major decisions. Use any and all resources to help you with this process but, above all, create a medical team for yourself that you trust.

Communications
You may choose to share your diagnosis with family and friends.

Suggestion: Consider creating an e-mail folder, maybe with subcategories, depending on the type of information:

- Kind e-mails from friends and family
- Cancer information
- Diet/Exercise health information
- Websites you find helpful
- Inspirational notes

Suggestion: Consider Caring Bridge website or setting up an e-mail list of friends and family members that you want to keep in the cancer treatment loop. Communications can quickly become exhausting if you are responding to everyone individually. If it would be helpful to you, perhaps even a family member or close friend could coordinate the communications.

Time

Ask your doctors how quickly treatment decisions need to be made. Find out how much time you have to do the research. Many survivors, looking back, wished they had taken a little more time before making their treatment choices. Other survivors are happy with their choices and glad they acted quickly. Here again, everyone has different medical circumstances and different styles of doing things. There is no one right way to handle this. Know yourself and ask your healthcare professionals what time frame would be best for you.

Researching Your Cancer

Everything you learn will help you to solve your problems.
What you don't learn will cause your problems.
Warren P. Brown

Listen to all, plucking a feather from every passing goose, but follow no one absolutely.
Chinese proverb

Internet

Try to stay with reputable websites if you use the Internet. You may be researching your disease. You need accurate information.

You may decide that what you find online upsets you more than it helps you. Can you delegate this task? Could a family member or close friend do some of the legwork for you? Or, can you rely on other sources of information instead, perhaps your medical team?

Consider your social network

Ask friends and family and anyone you know who has been through the cancer experience about doctors (surgeons, radiologist, oncologist...). You will be assembling a medical team for yourself. Choose a team you can believe in. As I mentioned before, having a great team on your side will help you emotionally too.

Your emotional support

It may be helpful to talk to someone who can help you with the onslaught of emotions too. Consider an oncology talk therapist and a cancer support group. If you aren't ready for this, that is okay too. This is all about what is most helpful to you right now, so you can make the best decisions and choices for yourself. You may also find it helpful to talk to one or more people further down the path that had a diagnosis similar to yours. They can offer a heartening perspective and a message of hope and survivorship.

Tool: Finding the Positives (yes, there *are* positives)

Change your perspective. The sooner you start looking for the silver lining, the sooner you can help yourself begin to feel better. Find the positives and write them down. I wrote about the benefits of my breast cancer (yes, Virginia, there is a Santa Claus, and there are some benefits) about 19 months out from diagnosis as a letter back to my newly diagnosed self:

Dear Self,

You do not realize it yet, but cancer will teach you so many things about interpersonal relationships, personal growth, spiritual change, acceptance and appreciation of life, concern for others, and health habits, among other things.

You will learn that you are truly blessed by your marriage. You will learn how much you love your husband and how much he loves you. He can't "fix" your breast cancer, but he can be by your side and comfort you tremendously. You will learn how kind people can be, including people who you didn't know very well before the diagnosis. You will be touched by the love and support that reaches out to you.

Oh, Self, you will learn that the days do add up, chemotherapy has an end-date (at least for now), and that you can get *through* this! You will get better at living in the moment, appreciating the small things and, dare I say it— learning patience!

You will also learn ways to deepen your faith and renew your spirit. You will read your Bible more. It will mean more to you than it has meant before, and even make a little more sense.

You will learn to take better care of your physical and emotional self, and you will learn that you truly have a spiritual self that is above, beyond, and behind your mental, physical, and even very emotional self! You will learn to exercise and eat better! You will be rewarded by a body that is actually healthier in many ways than you were before your devastating diagnosis. You will also grow in compassion and in your ability to reach out and love others who are struggling with things in their own lives. In short, this will be a time for you to grow.

By the time you are 19 months out from diagnosis (now), you will not be done growing. You will better accept that the cancer experience is a process and be more willing to give yourself the time you deserve to work through the process. You aren't alone, Self, the self-beating is done, and I've got your back!

There is a line from the movie *Steel Magnolias* that I truly love: "Beginnings are scary. Endings are sad. It is what is in the middle that counts."

Tools for Getting through Active Treatment

You Are in the Middle of the Fray

Keep in mind, at all times, that we grow the most from our greatest suffering.

As we go through it, it hurts.

But as we move through it, it also heals.

When a jug of water falls to the floor and cracks, what was hidden within begins to pour out.

When life sends you one of its curves, remember that it has come to help crack you open so that all the love, power and potential that have been slumbering within you can be poured into the world outside you.

And, like a fractured bone, we do become stronger in the broken places.

Robin Sharma

Maybe it is out of order to talk about time and progress at the beginning of your cancer survivorship journey. I will because I wished I had been aware of the true progress and wonder of time passing earlier in my own journey. That said, maybe it is a message that is hard to *hear* at the beginning and easier to *believe* later on. I have to try, for your sake. Here goes.

Every minute or hour or day, good or bad, under your belt counts and moves you forward through your cancer journey. Every time you can focus for even a few *moments* on something other than your cancer, it is something to celebrate. Your focus will change over time. Cancer will not always take over your brain every waking minute of every day. A fellow survivor shared that thought with me when I was in the middle of my treatment and it really helped. I clung to that thought and hope. She was a survivor looking back on her treatment journey and someday I hoped I would be looking back at this difficult window of time too.

That said, a cancer journey is a marathon and not a sprint. It may be a short or long course of treatment, but it is measured in weeks or months. It is not *forever*. Really. Recognize that it will take a chunk of time, but it is a *limited* chunk of time.

Here are several of my journal snippets at different points in time:

November 6

Can I live with the loss of certainty for the rest of my life (as my oncology therapist put it)? Can I create a "new normal"? What if I can't? I feel so overwhelmed, buried, and I have no energy or focus right now. The holidays are here. And, I am behind, behind, behind. The good news is that I have been sleeping. I am remembering a dream every night, and I think that's good because I must be getting to REM sleep again, finally.

December 21

Today I did 3 miles *Walk Away the Pounds*. I brushed the dogs, cooked the squash, and did some vacuuming. I met my friend Arvilla for lunch and we visited for a long time. More normal is feeling pretty good. Sometimes I feel like I can create normal for those around me better than I can create it for me. Other times, I feel like I am on my way there too. The dogs were not good this evening when we took Sarah to her bassoon lesson. They opened and ate the Christmas presents under the tree (including a hardcover book, some candy, some microwave popcorn, and wax candles, seriously!). We took pictures, laughed (a little), and then cleaned up the mess and the dog barf... What else?

My left hip aches a little, especially when exercising. I don't know if this is a side effect of the Anastrozole, a result of more exercise, or, frighteningly, cancer?

January 9

I did 2 miles *Walk Away the Pounds* with Dan. He made coffee. It was nice to sit and hang out together at breakfast. When I was going through treatments, I didn't see an "end," but now I see moments of a new normal and, regardless how long it lasts, I am grateful. I am grateful for each day as they come one by one. Dare I say it? Sometimes I feel happy. Other times, I feel buried by "new normal" life and I get stressed.

The chronological order of those entries above makes it look like I gradually improve. Well... yes and no. It is important to mention at this point that progress often isn't strictly linear or steadily upward. It is a spiky, jagged, upward journey. There were emotional backslides or things that would push my buttons—some logical and some that were unexpected. Some things still, and probably always will push my buttons or catch me off guard unexpectedly.

As fellow survivor, my friend Happy, puts it: "It's not the big moments that get me, it's the goofy little things and I suspect you feel that too. You have to be patient with yourself and your body."

Patience never was my strong suit. I think my breast cancer journey has helped me work on developing that skill! See, *there are good things that will come out of this experience.* Hang in there. Get through the tough stuff, and you will see. You are not alone and there are skills and tools to help you.

Expand your toolbox and your skill set today. I went to a teen parenting class a few years ago. I remember the instructor was trying to add more coping skills to our teen parenting toolbox. He said something I will never forget: "If all you know how to do is hammer, then everything in your toolbox starts to look like a hammer. Let me teach you some other options." It may not feel like it now, but you have options and choices here—skills you can improve, tools you can add to your toolbox, and resources that are there to help you get through this.

Marathon Survival Tools

How do you eat an elephant? One bite at a time.
Author unknown

Try not to let your mind race weeks or months ahead right now. Try to stay in the moment and tackle each treatment event as it comes.

The cleaning and scrubbing will wait till tomorrow,
For children grow up, as I've learned to my sorrow.
So quiet down, cobwebs. Dust, go to sleep.
I'm rocking my baby and babies don't keep.
Excerpt from a poem by Ruth Hamilton

Prioritize. Prioritize. Prioritize. This is a journey that will show you what is and isn't important in your life. Maybe it will be what you expect. Maybe not. One fellow survivor friend talked about chemotherapy this way: She said that during chemotherapy, your energy level is low and very limited. She said it is like having only three or four quarters to spend each day, so choose carefully what you spend them on.

Belief-System Tools

Believe you can and you will.
Author unknown

When faced with a life crisis (yes, this certainly qualifies), it is helpful to remind yourself to go back to basics, *your* basics. The core things that make you who you are can be the backbone that you may feel is missing right now. For many of us, there are two tools in this category: faith and nature. Not everyone finds comfort in their faith or is comfortable with faith. Others find comfort in their connectedness to nature. In this book, I share how faith helped me, but if faith isn't a helpful topic for you, please feel free to skip this section and explore the next tools. If faith and/or nature are helpful to you, embrace them. Use them as tools to help yourself through this. Turn to them for comfort and to keep your boat afloat in this crummy, stormy sea.

November 6

I had a couple of personal epiphanies today: I have a spiritual self—a true me, behind the scary thoughts (mind) and feelings (emotions) and body (physical). I can get caught in thoughts or I can learn to let them go. I can live in fear or I can choose to live in hope. I am going to try to live in hope. Time will pass either way, and I want to spend my life in hope and in helping others, not in fearful thoughts and fear. We all have fears. It is how we handle them that can make a difference both in our own personal quality of life and how we affect those around us.

May 15

My oncology therapist said they are starting to study the near-death experiences in hospital emergency rooms. There are objects on high shelves near the ceiling that can't be seen from the floor. People with near-death experiences are coming back and telling staff what is on those shelves. Intriguing and promising! I find hope in this.

Hang on to your hope. Nurture your hope. Trust in your hope. You may be able to hang on to your hope through your faith. Surround yourself with quotes. Read. Listen. Pray.

Have faith

Trust the Lord with all your heart
and do not rely on your own understanding.
In all your ways acknowledge Him
and He will make your paths smooth.
Proverbs 3:5–6
(First shared with me by Grandma T, 25-year breast cancer survivor!)

Fairy tales are more than true;
not because they tell us that dragons exist,
but because they tell us that dragons can be beaten.
G.K. Chesterton

Remember what you believe. Pray. Pray. Pray. Talk to God. Tell him how you are feeling and ask for the healing, guidance, and hope that you want. Don't go it alone. Ask for family and friends to pray for you. You are not alone. Remember that. While you are at it, even though it takes a lot of energy, call your pastor or rabbi or spiritual guide. Let them know what is happening in your life and ask for their prayers too. I also found the daily meditations from the Proverbs 31 Ministries website to be helpful to me.

The phone call to my pastor was the best call I ever made. The pastor immediately connected me with another recently diagnosed breast cancer patient in our congregation. We became a special support group of two! Reach out to your faith community. Do not do this alone. Even if there doesn't happen to be someone currently walking your walk, you may find support in your faith community. Turn to baby steps and basics.

"'But what about you?' he asked. 'Who do you say I am?'"
Matthew 16:15 (NIV)

"He is my Hope…"
When we are in the midst of a catastrophic situation, we find ourselves clinging to hope. The smallest glimmer of hope keeps our eyes open and our heads held up.

When we are in the midst of a frustrating situation, we find ourselves clinging to hope. The smallest glimmer of hope keeps us looking beyond the disturbance.

When we are in the midst of our daily routines, we find ourselves clinging to hope. The smallest glimmer of hope keeps us believing for something more …
(From the article "A Ready Answer" by Holly Good, assistant to Lysa TerKeurst, Proverbs 31 Ministries)

God is my Hope too. Sometimes it is all we have in the face of cancer, other life problems not easily solved, and the great unknown.

Kate, my friend and fellow breast cancer survivor, brought me a beautiful little book called *Moments of Peace for a Woman's Heart: Reflections of God's gifts of love, hope, and comfort* the day she learned I had the same diagnosis that she had. I found immediate comfort in the short passages and thoughts arranged by topic. Sometimes, a big thick book with long chapters is just too much on top of what you are already coping with and this book's small segments may be just right.

When we met for lunch while we both were on chemo, Kate also brought me Sharon Callister's book *On Wings of the Dawn: A devotional book for women experiencing breast cancer and their supporters.* It was here I first learned in great detail how a fellow Christian woman with a breast cancer diagnosis felt and coped with what she felt on her breast cancer journey. I liked the biblical quotes interspersed with her experiences and observations. Our diagnosis and experiences weren't identical, but I found comfort.

Maybe it will also help to combine faith with music. I found myself turning to my local Christian radio station with new zeal. The lyrics in some of the songs resonated with me in ways they hadn't prior to my breast cancer diagnosis. You could also download tunes that are helpful. Try the song "Blessings" by Laura Story. I really identified with some of her words.

Nature Tools

Live your life each day
as you would climb a mountain.

An occasional glance
Toward the summit
Keeps the goal in mind,
But many beautiful scenes
Are to be observed
From each new vantage point.

Climb slowly, steadily,
Enjoying each passing moment;
And the view from the summit
Will serve as a fitting climax
For the journey.
Harold V. Melchert

Remember your connectedness to the world, the Earth, or Nature. You became part of Nature and the world when you were born. It is your birthright. Nothing, not even cancer, can disconnect you from it, weather permitting, and even if the weather is bad because you can still look out a window.

You are part of the glory that is this world. Step outdoors several times a day and contemplate that. If the weather doesn't permit that, sit and look out a window. It is as simple as that. It is as glorious as that. Nature can anchor you and help you focus your attention away from your troubles.

Tie yourself into Nature and its rhythms and experience. It will help take you outside of yourself for precious moments that will give you a break from your health crisis. Center yourself with Nature. Meditate on the sights or sounds of Nature.

When you are outside or inside by a window, pick a sense and use it: catalog what you see, list what you hear, think about what you feel on your skin and under your feet, or notice smells. Being mindful of these things will help pull you into the moment and stop your mind from racing ahead with frightening thoughts.

Maybe you don't believe me? Get your upset self outside or to the window. Intentionally try it for five minutes several times per day for five days before telling me it doesn't help. You can try this.

People-Support Tools

Life is all about people helping people. Don't shut out anyone who wants to help you. They may not totally "get it" in terms of understanding what you are experiencing, but they care about you and want to help. Be grateful for this and let them help. Don't expect them to be psychic or to read your mind. Ask those around you for what you want or need.

If there aren't people you are close to, it may be time to make some new connections or to reconnect or repair some old connections. Failing that, there are other tools here. We have all had times of loneliness in our lives.

Family

I was a very fortunate person in that my family was invaluable during breast cancer treatment. I may have been upset, anxious and afraid, but I never felt unloved. My family unconditionally loved me and did what they could to "be" with me and support me through this experience. Other survivors talk about the importance of the help they got from a parent/spouse/partner/sibling. Still other survivors mention their support came from a "family" that they created instead of the family that they were born with.

Friends

A good friend is a connection to life:
A tie to the past, a road to the future,
The key to sanity in a totally insane world.
Lois Wyse

This might be a switch for you. Instead of being a friend to your friends, it is time to let those friends be there for you. Friends can help connect you with oncologists and other doctors *and* with fellow survivors! (Yes, every moment since your diagnosis, you are a survivor. Believe it.) As often happens with major life crises, some friends step forward the way you always thought they would, some don't, and others that you didn't expect to do anything help you more than you would have dreamed. I was grateful and appreciative of all kindnesses, large and small.

You may want to use the Caring Bridge website, or you may not. In my mind, I wasn't ready for Caring Bridge so I chose to create an e-mail group to get information out to concerned family and friends quickly. Some people ask a family member or good friend to take over communications. This is about doing whatever form of communication works best for you and fits your comfort level. It is helpful to figure out a way to get updates out to the people in your life without creating undue fatigue, stress or difficulties for yourself right now. You already have plenty to manage.

Professionals

Therapists: There are actually oncology therapists — talk therapists who specialize in helping cancer patients. Who knew? I hadn't been aware of them before my own diagnosis. I was extremely grateful to be referred to an excellent oncology therapist. It helped to be guided by someone who had helped other cancer patients. She had excellent understanding and advice. In addition, she validated my feelings and could talk, if I asked her, about how other cancer patients handled the practical or emotional issues that come up during and after active treatment.

Depending on your area, there may or may not be a talk therapist that specializes in cancer patients. Also, you don't always find a match or a fit with a talk therapist on the first try. Above all, if you want a talk therapist to discuss your cancer, make sure that person is a fit for you, and don't be shy about switching therapists if you don't have the fit you want.

Cancer support group: Find a support group. Find a support group. Find a support group. Yes, this was important enough for me to say at least three times. If you can't find one in your area, seriously consider making the drive to connect with one in a nearby community. That said, just like the right talk therapist, it is important to find a group where you feel comfortable and safe and supported. If a group doesn't have the right feel for you, it may not be the group for you. If you just don't like the idea of a support group, that is okay too—please feel free to skip to the next section.

If you can't find a support group or it is too far away, seriously consider creating a support group. It might only be a support group of two, but it would still offer benefits that aren't available if you choose to "go it alone." There are literally no words to adequately describe the emotional support generated by a room of people going through something very similar to what you are experiencing.

When I sit in my group, there is an hour or two of peace, whether I participate a lot or not, just from being with a group of people who "get it," and who fundamentally understand what I am experiencing. This doesn't even begin to touch on the emotional experience and also the informational experience of being part of a support group. Don't give up being part of a support group without a fight.

Don't do this alone. Repeat: Don't do this alone. There are many kinds of cancer support groups—breast cancer, Christian cancer support groups, general cancer support groups, family cancer support groups, and more.

If you can, shop around. Different groups have different leaders and different "vibes." Find one that is a fit for you, but don't give up on a group after one "bad" meeting either. Sometimes the tone can change from one meeting to the next. Take any medical information that you hear with a grain of salt because you are not a doctor and you don't know another cancer patient's medical history or complete story.

Oncology doctors: Again, find the right fit for you. You now are creating or have created a team of doctors. You may have an oncology surgeon, a medical oncologist, a radiation oncologist, a vascular specialist, and your regular doctor and perhaps others. Tell the doctors what you are feeling. If they don't know what you are experiencing, they can't help you. They are busy addressing the medical side of cancer and they aren't psychic. What you share won't be new to them, and they will have helpful suggestions (support groups, therapists, medications) for you to help you address things like sleeplessness, stress, and anxiety.

Oncology nutritionists: An oncology nutritionist can help with your eating choices during treatment and afterwards too. Learn what you can eat to fight back at cancer every day! My nutritionist explained what foods were "safe" during and after chemo, and gave me nutritional guidelines for calories, protein, fiber, fruits and vegetables, fluids, and more. Her advice has enabled me to make many better eating choices than I had prior to my first cancer diagnosis.

Physical therapists: A physical therapist will help you with regaining range of motion, reducing lymphedema and post-surgery swelling, and help to resolve other types of problems. Physical movement and exercise matter. Exercise improves mental health too. More on diet and exercise later.

Organizations

There are many organizations out there, especially when you have access to a computer and the Internet. My suggestion would be to stay with the more credible, large, readily recognized mainstream organizations—even some of them have their share of difficulties and bad publicity. I say this to help you protect your emotional self, not limit your options. If you find a conflict of information or emotionally upsetting post on a small blog or obscure discussion board, you may find that it does more emotional harm than good. As in all things, this decision is your own personal choice.

Here are some of the larger cancer organizations and their websites:

- American Cancer Society (ACS): http://www.cancer.org/
- American Institute for Cancer Research (AICR): http://www.aicr.org/
- National Cancer Institute (NCI): http://www.cancer.gov/
- The Mayo Clinic: http://www.mayoclinic.org/
- WebMD: http://www.webmd.com/
- LiveStrong: http://www.livestrong.org/
- Susan G. Komen: http://ww5.komen.org/
- Dr. Susan Love: http://www.dslrf.org/breastcancer/

Try not to wear yourself out over-researching. If you can, ask a friend or family member to hunt down answers to some of your questions that can be researched on the Internet. Remember to make lists of questions for your doctors too.

Calming Tools

Fall seven times. Stand up eight.
Japanese proverb found in Healthy Reflections, November 12, 2011 at SparkPeople.com

Do you wonder if you will ever feel "calm" again? Please try to trust that it will happen. There are tools that can help you. The trick is to keep trying things until you figure out what helps you the most. An oncology therapist can help be a catalyst and guide for positive change from this experience and help create a "new normal" for you. A "new normal" does await you. You will get there. Here are some tools to help:

Focus on the present

Your mind may want to race around and leap forward in time. To calm yourself, focus on the present—minute by minute, hour by hour, one day at a time. Don't look too far ahead. Above all, don't let worry carry you too far into the future.

Focus on the senses

Pick a sense (sight, sound, or touch) and use it to soothe yourself. Take a deep breath (or two or three), pick a sense, and spend a few minutes several times per day focusing on that sense, especially at times when you feel especially distraught or overwhelmed or shaky. Step outside to do this if you can.

I would often choose sight or sound outside when my brain would get too stirred up and upset. I would stand or sit outside for several minutes and continually pull my mind back to experiencing and listing the sights or sounds around me right at that moment. It was a simple exercise, but practiced consistently, it worked. It calmed and soothed me and got me through yet another window of time.

Sometimes in bed, I would close my eyes and focus on the funny shapes and colors floating under my eyelids. Other times, I would concentrate on listening and listing all the sounds I could hear inside and outside (the sound of traffic, the ceiling-fan chain clicking, the fan motor, the furnace blower, the creaking of the house).

Tactile distraction

Get something in your hands. Repeat: Get something in your hands. This can be a simple but huge help to provide some relief. My friend Kate went instinctively to crocheting. After treatment, she confessed that she had made over 14 afghans during active cancer treatment. She said she sometimes changed colors randomly. They weren't meant to be pretty, necessarily. She said she worked on them on her couch, in bed, in the car, at the lake…

Being a slow learner, I didn't catch on to this technique until close to the end of my radiation. I am typically not a crafts person, which might be compounded by the fact that I am a lefty.

I went on the Internet and found videos that demonstrated very basic crochet stitches. Scrunching the yarn in my hands felt good. Learning the stitches, and even shopping for yarn helped to redirect me from cancer fears and worries. Counting stitches row by row was extremely calming and distracting. I was amazed and wished I had tried it sooner. I also did some beading and bead making.

Other distractions

I tend to be from the "do-what-works" school of thought. Here are some more things to try.

Focus on a hobby: One of my good escapes was making paper beads at the kitchen table with one of my daughters. I was fortunate that my neuropathy wasn't bad, so I could do this. The bead making required a lot of fine motor skill and attention to detail. I was amazed that time could actually fly while working on beads with her.

Shopping and browsing: Why? Shopping is very outward and visual. Shopping helped draw me out of my circular negative internal thoughts. I liked going to antique stores because there was lots of sensory stimulation there, but for me as a non-antique collector, there was very little I would actually be tempted to buy. But, truth be told, almost any shopping or browsing was helpful to distract me. There was a caveat. Once I shopped at the local grocery store and ran into several neighbors and church friends. Their kindness and support was wonderful but exhausting. Later, I learned that sometimes women with breast cancer avoid church or shopping at their local store during treatment because of the chance of running into people who are concerned about them. It really depends on what you need at any given moment.

Television: There is a reason why there is one in every hospital room and the hospital televisions often have DVD players there too. Figure out what kind of shows help you and what kind don't, and then go for it! I found I needed to stay away from blood and gore shows, but well-written, humorous television series or comedy movies could be very distracting.

Audio CDs: There are a wide variety of options here including free smartphone applications. Categories to consider include New Age music, relaxation, meditation, and guided imagery to heal, relax, or sleep. Actively listening can be a helpful distraction, especially if watching television gets old.

I found my list of the things that personally calmed and soothed me and included it below. As I reached the end of chemotherapy and radiation, and my body and mind were really weary and exhausted, it helped me to look at this list for ideas. I could find something after a sleepless night or emotionally exhausting day that helped me. You may get some ideas from my list, but you may find it even more helpful to create your own personal list as you go and refer to it as you move forward.

Things that comfort or soothe me during breast cancer treatment

- Being with my husband
- Being with my daughters
- Being with my friends
- Talk therapy
- Being in my breast cancer support group because everyone around me "gets it"

- Petting my dogs
- Going outside and seeing, hearing, and/or smelling with every ounce of my being
- Listening to music
- Reading
- Watching light entertaining television
- Watching a good movie—clever and entertaining (not dark or bloody, please)
- Weeding and watering the plants
- Beading with a daughter
- Shopping and running errands with a daughter
- Shopping or browsing as a distraction
- Guided imagery and positive affirmation chemo tape and other meditation tapes
- Mundane household work when I have the energy
- Weeding out clutter when I can't sleep at night
- Crocheting! Who knew? It *is* comforting to squish the yarn in my hands and focus on concentrating and the tactile sensations of the task.
- Reading the gratitude list one of my daughters (Sarah) made for me on an especially tearful day

Self-Care Tools

Do not allow worry to take over your heart.
Heidi Ganzer, oncology nutritionist

I believe that anyone can conquer fear by doing the things he fears to do, provided he keeps doing them until he gets a record of successful experiences behind him.
Eleanor Roosevelt

Journaling

Write. Write. Write. For me, journaling is often all about getting thoughts and feelings from spinning around in my head and down on paper or computer. Cancer generates a lot of thoughts and feelings. Get them out of your head! You don't have to carry them all around with you all the time. Let a journal be a tool, not an anchor. That is, write when you feel like writing. Don't write when you don't want to write. You may write several times in a journal one day and then walk away from it for several days. Simply begin the top of each entry with the current date. Write what you think. Write what you feel. Write what you are observing and learning. Write what is hurting you. Write what you know.

List making

My brain felt overloaded by my breast cancer diagnosis. Stress is real. Chemo brain is real, and anyone who tells you otherwise isn't up on current research. That said, you may or may not have symptoms of chemo brain. I felt overwhelmed. Thoughts flitted in and out of my head, but I couldn't seem to hang on to them in an organized fashion. Lists are another way to download what is cluttering up your mind. Make lists of your fears, worries, and concerns, as well as practical things like questions for doctors or pharmacists, to-do lists, shopping lists, and planning lists.

Healthy eating—with your doctors' approval

(*There may be restrictions and suggestions depending on chemotherapy, radiation, or other treatments.*)

Healthy eating is a journey, not a single number on the scale. Does that help a little? This approach allows you to allow your body to fluctuate. Healthy eating is a much better term to regularly contemplate than all the negative connotations that go with a word like "diet." Why work on healthy eating? For me, there were several good reasons based on things I had read:

- Maintaining a healthy body weight may reduce the chances of cancer recurrence by as much as 40–70% depending on which study you are reading. Why isn't this being shouted from the rooftops? Here is a very clear and proven way to improve your own odds of staying healthy!
- Healthy eating helps with weight loss and cancer prevention. Think about antioxidants. Also, frankly, I needed to lose some weight.
- Mental health may be improved with healthy eating and stable blood sugars. I needed mental health to fight my cancer too.

Exercise—with your doctors' approval

(*Again, this will depend on your kind, type and stage of treatment.*)
Exercise helps with weight loss and mental health. It is a very active way that I can fight back at cancer almost every day. When active treatment ends and doctors aren't watching every minute, it can be a frightening and isolating time. How is the cancer being fought? What if it comes back? Who will know? Exercise is a way to fight back every day. A healthier body has less chance of recurrence. Exercise is a weapon you can put in your toolbox and wield it against cancer every day. Think Xena Warrior Princess if you want!

One AICR statistic says 30–45 minutes of aerobic exercise per day can help reduce recurrence.

Exercise releases endorphins. Endorphins help fight anxiety and depression from the cancer diagnosis. Exercise can improve mental health. Sometimes it works as well or better than depression or anxiety medications, and it doesn't have the side effects that the medications may have.

Humor

Yes, I said humor. Watch for it and make note of it! Everyone's sense of humor is different. I still smile when I go back and read (or add) something to my humor list. Just starting a humor list (even if you only have one thing to put on it) will help you improve your mindset because at least you will start being more on the lookout for something that makes you smile or laugh during this journey. A humor list can help you shift your perspective on life. Let humor in. Let humor help you too.

Here is a list of humorous moments from my own journal:

Barb's Breast Cancer Humor (yes, I wish this list was longer)

1. After chemo, "just like getting braces off," I can eat sushi and blue cheese again! (My daughter Emily noted the parallel with removing orthodontia.)
2. Going through the breast cancer process, I will finally learn how to wear hats and scarves! (Emily told me this. PS: I also learned how to wear a baseball hat.)
3. My 18-year-old daughter could have wine with dinner in Wisconsin because she was with her parents, but her mom couldn't because she was on chemo! (Or, at least, I chose not to drink.)
4. Ironically, the girl (me) who threw up in grade school through high school if she had to give a speech and who threw up when she broke up with a boyfriend in college, and who throws up when she is really emotionally stressed, *isn't* throwing up on chemo so far, so go figure.
5. When I am in a public place, like the mall, I am sometimes getting that up-down look by men where they check you out! Too funny! I am tempted to pull off my wig and tell them they are checking out an old, sick, bald woman with breast cancer! I guess this is a "payoff" for diet and exercise?!

6. When I cried in a restaurant to a girlfriend about the breast cancer stuff (discreetly according to her), the kind waitress brought us a dessert. Free dessert! Free *chocolate* dessert!

7. Dan (my husband) turned to me in the bathroom just the other day and asked me to get him some more of his hair-forming gel the next time I am in a hair product supply place. Like that will happen any time in the near future! Too funny! It will be months before I need hair supplies again.

8. Emily gave me an education and a beautiful quote when I lamented my near baldness: "Mom, now that you are slimmer, you can be like the models who deliberately shave their heads bald to draw attention to their beautiful bodies." My friend Pam made a comment about this too at lunch one day.

9. I discovered my favorite lipstick color in the world. It was in my ACS Look Good Feel Better freebie makeup! "Lucky" me! (I still wear and enjoy this color.)

A Personal Self-Help List

Here is a list of what personally helped me through breast cancer. It was helpful to write these ideas down and refer to my options when I needed them, especially the times I was too weary to come up with good ideas from scratch. Some of them came from people around me as you will see. I hope you consider making this list for yourself too! It may even be helpful to someone else you care about down the road… What supports you? In the midst of the chaos created by your diagnosis, what helps? When you are down, go look at your list and pick something to try.

My Self-Help Cancer Support List

1. Praying.
2. Reading the Bible.
3. Spending time with family.
4. Spending time with friends.
5. Cancer therapist.
6. Oncology nutritionist.
7. Breast cancer support group in my community.
8. Dragon Divas (breast cancer survivors who train and race dragon boats).
9. Reading breast cancer self-help books (some of them*).
10. Reading a devotional book.
11. Mp3 tapes. Guided imagery for chemo, for radiation, and for relaxation, also positive affirmation, self-hypnosis, subliminal, relaxation, and stress reduction tapes.
12. Regular exercise.
13. Healthful diet.
14. Hydration.
15. *Sleep* (when available).
16. *Doing something tactile like crocheting (I wished I'd "gotten" this sooner).*
17. Taking anxiety medications as frequently as prescribed.
18. Breathing exercise/meditation.
19. Picking a sense (auditory or visual), and focusing for several minutes only on that input (from Sandi T)—a few minutes every hour, building to maybe a half-hour once per day.
20. Doing something nice for someone else.
21. Petting the dogs.
22. Going outside.
23. Listening to music.
24. Reading for fun, specifically, books with happy endings.
25. Watching entertaining light television.

26. Watching a good movie—clever and entertaining (not dark or bloody).
27. Weeding and watering the plants.
28. Beading with Sarah.
29. Shopping and running errands with Emily.
30. Shopping as a distraction.
31. Working on book promotion activities when I have the energy.
32. Mundane household work when I have the energy.
33. *Letting go of my expectations* (Laura). Drop all "shoulds" and "oughts" right now. Another survivor, Sandy G, said the eleventh commandment could be "Thou shalt not shouldeth thyself."
34. Force yourself to do one of the activities above until you can come back in a different place (tip from Laura). *Distraction.* Anything to get out of your own head.
35. Postpone the tough stuff (write it down if you need to) until you have more resiliency to deal with it (tip from Laura).
36. Remind yourself that a lot of this isn't really you: the treatment has you. You don't have to take your emotions seriously or own all of them at this point in time. The emotions are hijacked by the cancer treatment for the time being.
37. I don't have to get an "A" in cancer treatment. It is not a competition. I just have to get *through* it.

*Some books helped. Some didn't. The ones that didn't help me had conflicting information about what to do about my breast cancer or frightened me. If a book cites too many scary stories or creates conflicting thoughts or fears, consider putting it down. You can always get back to it when you are further down the road, if you want. Don't dwell on the negative. Not right now.

Hanging Loose

Here is my analogy: humans as hot-air balloons. We plan a route, trying to take weather and wind into consideration, but the wind and weather changes and life doesn't always happen the way we predict it will. Intellect is the pressurized propane tank and burner. Emotions are the flame that heats the air in the balloon. The soul or spirit is the unseen air inside the balloon that shapes the balloon. The ballast is the baggage and experience we carry, intellectual and emotional, needed or not. The wind is God. We can float. We can observe. We can slightly alter our course—direction, speed, how high we choose to fly. We don't have to engage. We can be flexible. We aren't in control—even with our blowers and flame and plans (intent). Not being in control doesn't mean we should quit trying or planning. It just suggests that we might be happier and more effective if we can be flexible.

Attachment can be good and bad. Attachment to positive thoughts, choices and people and experiences is helpful. We can cling to them during this chaotic time.

Attachment can also be negative. Attachment to things we can't control can hurt. I think happiness and peace exist in the moment. There is comfort in familiar surroundings and "stuff," yet vacations can be exhilarating, freeing, and exploratory. We don't freak out when we go on vacation. We anticipate, explore and, in one way or another (photos, souvenirs, ideas), we try to bring something from our experience back home.

Hindsight

The excursion is the same when you go looking for your sorrow as when you go looking for your joy.
Eudora Welty

Hindsight is always 20-20 (or better). Looking back can provide an insight and clarity that is difficult to have when you are caught up in the middle of an experience. I worked on this list as I began to learn things on this journey. This is probably no news flash, but the truth is that I am still learning and adding to the list below.

Insights that I wish I had known at the beginning of my breast cancer journey (the list below came from my personal journal. I hope you can learn from my mistakes, and make your journey a little more comfortable or doable as a result):

Cancer stuff I would handle differently (hindsight always being 20-20)

- I would be kinder to myself. Much kinder.
- I would go to people who comfort me, not push them away.
- I would be more regular about taking full doses of prescribed medications for the anxiety, stress, and sleep issues.
- I would crochet and squeeze the yarn more or keep my hands busy with any craft or activity.
- I would pet my dogs and draw comfort from moments with them.
- I would meditate and/or focus on the external senses more.
- I would make a deliberate effort to read the Bible every day, for me.
- I would remind myself that I can cry and be brave all at the same time.
- I would strive to hold in my mind the realization that active treatment is a limited-amount-of-time process.

What would cancer survivors want to tell those who love us? How can loved ones help us?
The letter below is what I wish I could have explained to the people who were there for me at that time:

Dear Friend/Family/Caregiver,

I am grateful you are here, especially now. You may be feeling sad, worn out, stressed, or worried that you don't know how to help. Please believe me when I say that just being here with me is a huge comfort. I know you can't solve this cancer or make it go away.

Sometimes I just want you to listen and be with me. Be with me in this place. Please just *be quiet* and listen. That is so kind and helpful of you. When you speak, don't worry about saying the wrong thing. Whatever comes out of your mouth won't make the cancer worse.

Hold my hand or give me a hug if you wish. I am not contagious. I am very alone at times. Physical contact is a blessing. If it doesn't feel good, I will move away or let you know.

Please don't let cancer be the elephant in the middle of the room. If I am happy, please be happy with me. If I am sad, you can be sad with me too. Please just *be* with me. Please ask or say whatever comes to you. Asking me about it is not going to hurt me or make me sad. I am with the cancer 24-7. You won't be suddenly reminding me about something I have forgotten. I wish that were the case!

KS, a fellow survivor, shared these thoughts:

My best advice is always "Make a plan." Remembering my diagnosis, hearing "You have cancer" is three little words you don't want to hear. Once heard, you crumble, cry, panic... and then some well-meaning nurse tells you she can get you in to see the doctor in two weeks! *No!* You and your support team need to get a plan in place. Once you have a plan on which you can execute, you will take back control of this diagnosis and get back in charge. I have shared this advice with other women and they agree. We like to be in control, we take charge and with this diagnosis, that is briefly taken away from us. Make a plan, execute on the plan, stay on the plan. This is your life, your schedule, your plan.

The other advice I would like to share is: Take care of the caregivers. Now that I have been through the experience, my passion, support, gifting, and time is all spent on caregivers. No one walks this path alone. If you are well and healthy, reach out to those who are taking care of others. Give them a call, thank them, drop off a small basket of lotions, candles, relaxing items. Caregivers don't complain, they lose sleep too, they keep the world turning. We owe them a great debt of gratitude.

What would caregivers and people who have loved and helped cancer patients want to tell the caregivers and loved ones of newly diagnosed cancer patients?

Caregiver/daughter/wife AC shared:

The most important things that I learned helping both my parents deal with multiple types of cancers was to remind them that they are loved and that they are not alone in this fight. A person going through cancer treatment needs to know that they have loved ones and friends that are there for them who will do whatever needs to be done to help them get through the treatments and that after all that is done and their bodies have a chance to recover from the drugs and radiation, they will have a life to live once again. That life will never be the same and they will have to make changes in their lives to meet the new goals they set for themselves, but there is a light at the end of the long hallway that they have been walking through.

You sometimes need to be the mean one who pushes them to go to treatment even though they will feel sick after, with the hope that in the long run they will come back to themselves and to us. We need to let them know that we understand they do not feel well but we cannot just let them give up and sit around thinking negative thoughts and just giving up the fight, because there is a light at the end of it all and that light is being able to start again, maybe with different goals, and they will look at life in a different way than they did before the cancer, after realizing that there is more to life than getting the promotion or a bigger house; it is friends and family that love you and need and want you around. These people who will lose a very important part of themselves if you give up and do not fight for your life.

I found that, with my parents, just talking to them daily about what was happening in my life gave them something else to think about other than the cancer and the treatments. It gave them something to look forward to, finding out how their grandson was doing in Boy Scouts, at school and about what he and the dog did to get in trouble that day. I also found that keeping their minds on things other than their cancer and its treatment helped them to deal with the issue. I got my father out walking daily with the dog and he visited with the neighbors as he walked around the block. I got my mother doing crafts, latch hooking rugs which she made into pillow and wall decorations, and making artificial flower arrangements which she gave to friends. I also took my parents out to dinner and just running errands with me to get them out to see that the world was still out there and that there was a reason to fight and get back into it. *Do not* let your loved one just sit around the house and worry about the cancer, surfing the Internet looking at all the information out there, because it will then consume their minds and their lives and they will start to feel that it is hopeless and that too many things can go wrong or it could spread.

Now my experience was with my parents, mother had breast and colon cancer, father had colon and stomach cancer, and later in life my brother had stomach, colon and liver cancer. Every cancer type is different in their treatment and effect on the person, so my experience may not be the same as yours, but the main thing that is always true is that *they need to know that they are loved and their presence in our lives is important and that giving up is not a good option.*

My friend LH wrote:

I have not had breast cancer, yet. I do not know what a person who is dealing with the diagnosis is going through. I do not know what a breast cancer survivor is going through. I am just a friend who gets to stand by the sidelines on the journey, and support as best I can.

It is a journey the person walks by themselves. No one else can walk it with them. I cannot take the pain, fear, or depression away. However, I can try to make moments better when my friend is ready for that.

The best thing I can do is listen. Really listen. As best I can, offer a space where my friend can talk. As a friend, I have not heard all she can say. I am not her significant other who may have heard repeatedly what she is going through. And if she wants to repeat what she has told me many times over, that is okay.

So, as best I can, I listen. No interruptions, no questions, no ideas that come from me, no opinions or judgments, no helpful hints. If I talk, it may turn out to be more about my story, my feelings, my thoughts, and this time is for her, not me.

It may sound easy, but it is not necessarily easy. Because this journey is a tough journey that my dear friend is going through, and I really can't take the pain away. So, to be the best listener, I need support from my friends and family to make sure my needs are met in other ways. I do this so that when I am with my friend with cancer *I can listen to my friend with my best attention and intention.* So, I make sure I am rested, fed, and listened to by someone else.

I am going to mention some of the advice that is in the article "6 Things Not to Say to Someone with Depression" by Lindsay Holmes (*Huffington Post*, posted January 29, 2014). I mention it because it rings true to me in many situations. There are many things we say with the best intentions that really end up not validating or supporting our friends. Some of those things include: "I know how you feel," "Suck it up," "Cheer up," "Just think, others have it worse than you."

I don't know how a breast cancer survivor feels. I have never had breast cancer. If I did, then the phrase might be comforting (you are not alone; what you feel is normal). But I can't know what she feels. Also, even if I had breast cancer, each journey is different, and my journey is definitely going to have some different twists and turns than my friend.

Tears are not comfortable for most of us to be around. Over the years, I have learned to be much more comfortable with tears. They are a good way to release all the things that are bottled up. Often, after a good cry, a friend can think clearer and feel better. It is rare to have a safe place to cry. If you can let your friend cry, and be relaxed about it, that can be a gift. In contrast, I find when people say to me things like "Suck it up," "Cheer up," or "Others have it worse than you," what they are telling me is "Stop feeling this way because you make me uncomfortable." It is not safe to be vulnerable with them.

Daughter of a breast cancer survivor, EB shares:

Being a caregiver is difficult. It is hard to go from the one being taken care of, to the one taking care. Take each day as it comes; no two days will be the same. Never forget to care for yourself. Make time to decompress, feel and be present. In my case, my mom never asked for anything so it was important that I anticipated her needs.

If her water was getting warm, instead of asking her if she wanted me to refill it, I would just do it. Always remember to follow your instincts; if something doesn't seem right call the nurses. That is what they are there for. There is no need to suffer during treatments. If the person you are caring for is suffering, call the nurses, they can help. And finally, stay positive. Positivity can go a long way, for both your own spirit and for those around you.

Tools for Survivorship after Active Treatment

Every day I can work on becoming the person my dog thinks I am.
Author unknown

Creating a "New Normal"

If you want to lift yourself up, lift up someone else.
Booker T. Washington

Count your blessings, not your stressings.
Author unknown

Take stock of where you are now. You have been through a lot. Give yourself all the time that you need to recover. I am talking about months and years here, not just days or weeks. Repeat: Months and years, not days or weeks. Give yourself time. Just because active treatment has ended doesn't mean your body can instantly reset itself. The treatments have taken their physical, mental, and emotional toll on you. Be patient and kind to yourself. Spend some time thinking about what "being kind to yourself" looks like. Include some of that in your daily life. Be gentle with yourself. Think about what you would do for a friend or suggest to a friend who has been through cancer treatment and do that for yourself. It is a little different for each of us. You know yourself best.

If you start to mentally beat yourself up for not coping better or being further along by now, try this: Imagine you are sitting across from a dear friend who has been through exactly what you have experienced and is beating herself up for the same things. What would you say to her? How would you comfort her? What would you suggest that she do?

Think about what you lost

Yes, there has been a loss, and it deserves to be and needs to be acknowledged and mourned. If you acknowledge and fully experience your losses rather than stuff them, you will have greater resolution of your experience. If you try to stuff or bury those feelings, they can come back and bite you or bubble up in weird ways.

Your feelings will gradually improve over time if you can be aware of them and allow them to be what they are. It is a deep and pervasive loss. Time will help heal this. Sometimes I personally have to think about today compared to a year ago. I look at my journal and I am amazed at the healing that has happened to me. I also mentally replay things that survivors who are "further out" have told me. I find courage and hope and strength in their words.

Think about what you have gained

Yes, I really said "gained." When I met with Dr. CC for a second opinion about a prophylactic surgery (to remove ovaries and uterus), one of the things she said to me was, "I want you to take this [breast cancer] experience and start thinking about the positives that have come from it. You may think I am crazy now, but a little bit down the road from now I want you to start to do that." I tilted my head at the time, but further down the road I did begin to see her point.

Here is a list from my personal journal of some of the personal positives that came out of this journey for me. I hope you consider creating a list like this for yourself too.

Good things that came from my breast cancer experience

1. Many of the kind talented people that I met—including Dragon Divas (dragon boat paddling breast cancer survivors).
2. The things I learned about myself and the family and friends around me.
3. Significant improvement in reducing my self-beating tendencies—life literally is too short for beating ourselves. (Thank you, Sandi, and yes, the timing to actually be able to hear that message is everything.)
4. Improved knowledge that emotions are, well, just emotions, and they don't define me (again, thank you, Sandi). I can cry *and* be brave, and I do and I am!
5. The realization (from my o.b./gyn. Dr. H) that part of the legacy I leave my daughters is how I handle breast cancer and breast cancer recovery. Like it or not, I am a role model, and I want to actively choose to be the best model for them that I can every day that I am here.
6. A stronger faith. Thank you, Lord.
7. Perspective: less effort on sweating the small stuff, for real, to the core of my being.
8. An improved ability to prioritize my life.
9. I discovered that I looked pretty cute in a hat.
10. I discovered that I look good with short hair!
11. I found my favorite shade of lipstick ever in the ACS Look Good Feel Better goodie bag! (Okay, this item is filed under the 'breast cancer humor list' as well as here.)
12. Hopefully a level of compassion and awareness of others' struggles that I didn't have before.
13. A greater appreciation for the wonderful little moments in life.
14. More enjoyment of the outdoors and my senses—sight, sound, and touch.

The list above is a list that I continue to add to as more time passes. Please don't be lazy: Don't just read my list. Create your own. You can do this! Good things will come to you from your experience and you will be better able to see and appreciate them if you take note of them.

Weave the cancer journey into the fabric of your life

The way I see it, if you want the rainbow, you gotta put up with the rain.

Dolly Parton

Think about who you were going into cancer, who you were during your treatment, and who you are becoming. It isn't safe to stick your head into the sand and pretend it didn't happen. It probably isn't wise or healthy to dwell or wallow forever in this life event either. Instead, try a middle-of-the-road or balanced approach to incorporating what happened to you into the rest of your life journey. Unfortunately, you may not know where the middle of the road is. That is normal too. Allow yourself to make mistakes as you try to figure out what balanced looks like for you.

My friend Julie who leads a terrific breast cancer support group that has lasted many years says she has never met a person who has gone through this experience and not come out the other side as a stronger, braver, and wiser woman!

Here is my own running list of my personal changes. I wonder what yours will look like?

- Think healthier
- Eat healthier
- Exercise more
- Sweat the small stuff less
- Prioritize better
- Be grateful more often

People Support Revisited

Remember, we all stumble, every one of us. That's why it's a comfort to go hand in hand.
Emily Kimbrough, from "Shining Your Light on a Friend's Shade", Healthy Reflections, August 5, 2011 at SparkPeople.com

What do you need now that active treatment has ended? The answer may vary depending on whether you are months or years out from active treatment or somewhere in-between. Once you start looking healthy again, the people in your life are happy for you and probably assume you *are* healthy again. This can be tough. Physically, you may still be recovering, and emotionally and mentally, you may still be recovering too. Sometimes you may find yourself in a place where you aren't thinking about cancer every moment, and you would like to stay in that wonderful place for as long as you can. Other times, you may want to talk about your anxiety, fears, worries, pending appointments, health issues that arise…

Take care of you. Do not expect people around you to be psychic. If you need to talk, you can ask: "I trust you as my friend and I have appreciated your support. Can we talk about my cancer for a few minutes?" By now you may have found new friends, perhaps fellow survivors or other friends in your life who "get it," and you have figured out which people in your life won't be able to deal with your cancer discussion in a way that helps you.

This is what I wrote ten months out from active treatment:

I am blessed and grateful to have a good social support network. As I have said before, my husband has been great. My daughters are loving teenagers… My parents have been struggling with their own health issues. My in-laws have been kind and caring. I was fortunate to have a couple of close friends who were willing to hang in there with me and allowed me the freedom to cry and to vent when needed. I was also lucky to make a couple of new friends that were insightful and kind during and beyond my active treatment. I see a therapist who specializes in oncology patients, and I am also in a breast cancer support group that meets monthly.

What do I need from my social support network? I am not sure. I think it is my responsibility to reach out to my friends and family when or if I need them. As for wishful thinking, I wish that someone, besides my husband, would sometimes take the plunge and inquire something like: "So, how is your recovery going? How are you feeling?" Am I looking for pity? I don't think so, but maybe? I am ten months out from active treatment so it still feels very current as far as side effects (joint pain, fatigue...) and it still is emotionally worrisome.

I think it is understandable that people don't ask. Everyone is busy. I look "normal." And they probably think asking about my cancer could be a painful reminder to me. I don't know. I used to feel that way too, but then we had a death in the family and I was appreciative of the people who asked and reached out. I learned not to be afraid to address something that is painful to someone. Just because no one talks about it doesn't mean that those who have been affected by it (whatever it is—illness or death) have magically forgotten it.

If people did ask, it would be nice because the ball wouldn't always be in my court. I would feel less like I was intruding on the people I love if I wasn't the only one who brought it up in conversation. It would feel like it would be more okay to talk about it if they sometimes asked me. Does that make sense?

How could I get people to ask? I guess I could ask them to inquire, but that just feels weird and like I am asking for pity. I think I just get to be an adult and to take responsibility for bringing it up when I need to bring it up.

Looking back on this entry, I think part of my emotional needs as I worked on "new normal" would have been helped by more frequent attendance at the breast cancer support group I joined. Some women there were members for years and there is at least one study that shows support group attendance can help quality of life for survivors.

Moving Forward after Cancer
(a work in progress day by day)

1. I am less afraid of everything else—everything that isn't cancer. Why worry about the small stuff?
2. The days are longer now. Every moment of every day that is cancer-free is a delight and a gift. Time stretches out and I enjoy the small stuff and the little moments.
3. *I hate cancer.* That being said, I contemplate how to fight cancer and help others. Anger by itself just isn't a productive response long term.
4. A choice: Dive back into "normal," or help fight the fight, or something in-between? Decide what direction or mix or balance works best for you. Allow yourself to change over time on this topic too.
5. I still fight cancer every day by making healthy eating choices and exercising.

Things I will try not to do again
(I am such a work in progress here)

1. Avoid making the effort to ask questions and comfort someone going through any kind of difficult time (health, death in the family, job, anything).
2. Place taking care of stuff (chores) ahead of taking care of people—including me!
3. Skip taking the time each day to focus on what the

priorities for the day really are.

4. Be mean or sarcastic back when a teenage daughter gets snotty or lippy.

5. Open my mouth when it is better if it just stays shut.

6. Say things that are petty or unkind.

7. Hurt a friendship by opening my mouth to make my own point.

8. Make selfish choices.

9. Be impatient or seek instant gratification.

A Word about October
(especially for breast cancer survivors)

Breast Cancer Awareness Month, otherwise known as Think Pink for October

Some breast cancer survivors relish this month and many others breathe a sigh of relief on November 1st. Your feelings about this month may change over time too.

Breast Cancer Awareness month, October, puts breast cancer too much, too often, and too intently in my face. Wherever I go, it seems inescapable this month. In the coffee shop, there are pink heart helium balloons and pink crepe paper decorations, a banner, posters, and an 8' table display selling coffee in bags decorated in, you guessed it, pink. There is stuff at the grocery store, drug store, restaurant, and billboards, everywhere. How much do we need to be reminded every day for a whole month?

Breast cancer is *not* the only cancer or life-threatening disease out there. There are too many other diseases and cancers. Other cancers and other diseases deserve the support, attention, and research dollars and efforts too. All the focus, for an entire month, on breast cancer alone doesn't feel fair to me and sometimes other survivors feel this way too.

If you already loved pink before a breast cancer diagnosis, I am happy for you. Personally, as I mentioned before, I have never been a fan of pink. I remember my childhood room had pink walls, pink carpet, a lamp with pink fringe, and I think a pink bedspread. Under the glaring overhead light bulb, it was too much. I was tired of pink before I was done being a kid.

My oncology therapist said many other breast cancer survivors feel the same way I do about the onslaught. I was happy to hear that. She said cross the days off the calendar for the month of October and then be happy when it is over. Some people come in to appointments wearing the paraphernalia, and others, like me, aren't such good sports about it. We each get to make our peace with this month in our own way.

Cancer touches many people. All cancers, all illnesses for that matter, deserve the attention and research dollars that breast cancer receives. That is one of the concerns I have with October. The other concern is how much of this is truly helpful and how much is a marketing ploy? Just how many cents of each dollar raised goes to fight cancer? The answer can vary widely from coffee to yogurt to soup, and from company to company. Be an aware and astute donor in October, and any other time for that matter. Is there a maximum threshold? How are the dollars spent? What percentage of each dollar goes to fight cancer?

If you are a breast cancer survivor or someone who lost a loved one to breast cancer, how do you feel about this annual onslaught of pink for one month? My first October out from active treatment, I had to put up blinders, pull my head down, and just get through it. Regardless of your reaction to this month, know that you are not alone and you will get through it.

Putting Away the Cancer Supplies
(for now)

Worry does not empty tomorrow of its sorrow. It empties today of its strength.
Corrie Ten Boom, author and human rights activist

Weeding out and throwing away the physical paraphernalia from a cancer journey is an emotional issue. You may choose to do it all at once. You may choose to revisit this several times. You may have done this weeks or months ago. You may not even have considered it yet. Sometimes clutter needs to come off in layers (*Clutter Clearing Choices* by Barbara Tako, O Books, 2009. Yep, I had to include my first book in this one). Sometimes you can make a clean sweep of cancer supplies all at once. There is no single "right answer" here or "one size fits all."

Maybe you have thrown away, given away, or stored some items after each stage of your journey—surgeries, chemo, and radiation. Maybe there are things still lingering in medicine cabinets, drawers, and closet shelves. There are points in this journey where you may not want the visual reminders around. There are points in this journey where their presence may be comforting.

Do you wonder if you should keep some of the supplies "just in case"? Do you feel superstitious about getting rid of everything? Or maybe you feel superstitious about keeping these items? It is your call. You may get to a point where even if you aren't ready to get rid of these things, you may not want to see them in your daily routine in your home. I wrote in my journal when I got to this point. I hope you find my story here helpful as you consider what your story will look like:

November 18
I want to put away my cancer stuff. I have a box on the upper shelf of my walk-in closet and a drawer in my chest of

drawers. The box literally looms over me from its high shelf corner every day. I want to work harder and more deliberately to move cancer to a back burner in my life. Having the paraphernalia around is a reminder. I wonder what other survivors do? Right now, for me, it feels like emotional clutter. Maybe at this point, I want to try a little "out of sight, out of mind" and see where that takes me. Today I bought a big plastic lidded container that I could store in an out-of-the-way place.

Many months ago I had weeded through my cancer stuff. I had passed some on to a friend who was diagnosed shortly after me. I think I threw out a few things too. This time there isn't much of anything to toss, but it is time for some relocation.

I cleaned out the "breast cancer" dresser drawer and repurposed it as a short-sleeve T-shirt drawer. I cleaned out the "cancer" box that had been looming over my head in the closet and turned it into a holiday gift storage box.

I combined all the pills with a little water and then I put it in the kitchen trash and took it out to the garbage, and I threw away all the empty pill bottles. (There are better ways to properly recycle unused medications now.) I gave one of my daughters the crocheted scarf I finished. I put the yarn, the partial scarf, and the crochet hook in with the craft supplies in the laundry room.

The thoughtful cards I received, the supplies for eyelashes and eyebrows, the wigs, and the breast cancer giftware, headbands, hats, jewelry, and tote bags went into the new storage bucket too. I also put away some of my Diva-wear and Race for the Cure T-shirts hanging in the closet—some went in my exercise drawer and some went into the storage bucket.

Right now, I don't want to see daily reminders hanging around in my closet and dresser drawers. I can't make what happened go away, but it doesn't have to be seen several times per day in my bedroom, in my home. Does that make any sense?

I still have my lymphedema sleeve, antibiotic travel pills, and exercise bra vests in my dresser. That is only common sense. I also have the jewelry and encouraging note that Mom sent me while I was having chemo, a pink breast cancer bracelet from my friend Arvilla, and a list about the things that cancer can't take away tucked in a dresser drawer I don't open very often. I moved the physical therapy exercise information sheets and the journal record of my treatment into the two very large breast-cancer folders that I already have in our file drawers. They need to be weeded out too, but this is enough for today. I know my limits.

Dan made spaghetti and meatballs for dinner. I decided to join my family in eating this with them—though I added a spinach salad and some dried fruit to their meal of spaghetti, bread, and pineapple. It was good to all sit at the kitchen table together. (I am supposed to be cleaning up right now.) Looking around the kitchen, it felt lighter and more normal to me even though there never had been any cancer paraphernalia in this room—unless I count the little glass bird Ruth gave me that sits on my windowsill by the Christmas cactus. To me, the little bird is just a cheery reminder of a new friend reaching out to me. There are no breast cancer logos on it, and it isn't pink! Oh, and my in-laws gave me the Christmas cactus after one of my surgeries last year, but when I look at it now, all I see is a large beautiful flowering cactus. Moving forward. Moving through this. Time to go clean up after dinner…

If you are not ready to take this step, that is completely fine. If you already took this step, good for you! Did you throw everything away or keep some kind words and supplies that were helpful? The choice is completely yours. You get to decide when and if weeding these things out from your daily routine is helpful to you.

Trusting Your Body Again?

The present is what slips by us while we're pondering the past and worrying about the future.
Ziggy, cartoon foible found in Healthy Reflections, November 11, 2011 at SparkPeople.com

Will it be possible to trust your body again? How long will this take? This section could have started something like: "It's only tennis elbow, really," as I drove home from the sports doctor in tears. I actually smiled when I realized I was upset about something that wasn't cancer, sort of… After I thought about it, it would have been surprising if I hadn't been upset:

I began today with a trip to the dermatologist. I was getting a discount on some cosmetic fixes in lieu of the dermatologist reducing the appearance of the breast cancer scars. She is a very kind soul. To my way of thinking, I was excited to have a chance to reduce some of the visible damage or aging my face took on during my cancer journey. It didn't turn out to be as "fun" as I thought. As it turns out, a trip to the doctor, any doctor, for any reason, can evoke post-traumatic stress disorder (PTSD) symptoms—sort of emotional memories from all the cancer doctor appointments. It makes sense. It just isn't much fun. I found myself holding my breath during her treatment of my face rather than being able to converse with her while she worked.

Later that afternoon, I had an appointment with a sports doctor. Again, I was actually kind of excited to go get my tennis elbow resolved. It was something that wasn't cancer! The oncologist had ordered an x-ray a couple of weeks back, and after months of elbow pain I had learned from the x-ray results that it wasn't bone metastasis. That was good news!

Unfortunately, I found out the best option for my

particular tennis elbow would be weeks of physical therapy. I had already tried that for several weeks for some low back pain that had gone on for a year and was now triggering a bone scan scheduled for next week—once again to rule out bone metastasis. In addition to the physical therapy for the elbow, they wanted me to ice (which I had already tried) and wear something on the lymphedema arm at night (another reminder that things "aren't right" as well as a possible danger to compress that arm). I passed on the armband and left the sports medicine office in tears with more instructions yet to follow. Once again, I wanted an instant gratification sort of answer, not more work, and certainly not more reminders. That isn't how dealing with health issues or moving on from cancer works. Grr.

As part of a cancer survivor study, I had written a letter to my body a few weeks before that. After what happened to me that day, it was helpful to me to reread it and I want to share it now with you:

Dear Body,
Wow. You have been through a lot in the last 19 months. Sometimes I forget that and I forget to give you credit for it, or I forget to cut you some slack when you need it (i.e. run out of energy).

I am sad for you on many fronts. I am sad about the scars (a daily reminder I see), the harsh chemicals and radiation you endured, and all the adrenaline and cortisol that I sent your way for weeks and months too. I am sad about the toll all this has taken on you.

I am afraid for you too. I am afraid of the cancer coming back. I am afraid of every ache and pain and the need for each one to be subjected to a cancer rule-out diagnosis ahead of everything else. I don't blame you, but I am not sure how much I can trust you, at least yet. I also am angry for both of us. I am angry that it happened. I am angry about the ongoing side effects when I want to move forward. Fear and anger feel like two sides of the same coin. I am learning to allow myself the anger, and also try to move beyond the anger to more productive responses. I am not there yet.

I don't blame you for getting cancer. I feel guilty, and sometimes I do try to blame myself. I wonder if I had eaten better or exercised more or drank less wine or alcohol or exposed you to fewer chemicals... It really bugs me that I don't know why you got cancer or what magic thing I could do to guarantee it won't come back. Sometimes having had cancer feels shameful—yes, they cut a lump out of me and, yes, my hair fell out. Maybe some of it was my fault? When I start thinking about it like that, I try to quit the self-beating, but it is hard.

There is thankfulness too. I am thankful for the sisterhood of women I am connected to—you all truly get it, the friends that have reached out, and I am thankful for a good prognosis (not perfect, but good). I am thankful that my diet and exercise habits are better. I am thankful for the weight loss and short haircut. You have hair! It is different hair, but, nevertheless, it is hair. You have smaller clothing, even compared to high school. That should be more fun than it feels like so far.

Love, I am working on loving you again, Body. That is a little hard without trust, but I hope I can improve over time. I hope we can move on from the hurt and move forward in health and in love. You look pretty good, so let's work on feeling good physically and emotionally and moving forward!

There has been a loss. It will take some time to mourn. It will take some time to improve trust. If trust in your body is an issue for you, realize that recovering or improving it could take months or years. Please give it time. Please take comfort in knowing that you aren't alone in having these feelings. Again, this is a normal response to an abnormal situation.

In addition to time, it takes some successes—test results and blood work and examinations that *don't* show cancer. As you learn that everything that can go wrong isn't always cancer, it may stir up those cancer feelings, but it may also help teach you on a gut level, an emotional level, that *not everything is cancer.* I wish just reading those words would resolve it for you but I go back, instead, to repeating: Give it time. Score some successes. It will get better.

One survivor also mentioned to me that for some women the breast cancer experience becomes a crutch. Maybe there was lots of help and attention during active treatment for the cancer but at some point, as things got better, the extra help and attention started to go away? Dealing with that can be a transition to work through too. Be patient and gentle with yourself. Try to move forward without pushing a lot of "shoulds" and "oughts" onto yourself.

Gratitude Tool

Pay attention when an old dog is barking.
Old proverb in "Learn from Someone Who's Been There", Healthy Reflections, October 24, 2011 at Sparkpeople.com

This story would not be complete without a discussion of gratitude and its importance in my life and, hopefully, yours. Even with a cancer diagnosis and perhaps, especially with a cancer diagnosis, it is helpful and vital to actively practice gratitude.

Contemplate what you have instead of what you have not.

Gratitude increases resistance to life's curve balls. It improves your outlook on life. Practicing gratitude can rewire your brain to see things more positively. Gratitude is a wonderful life-tool.

Here is an ongoing list I kept in my journal. I hope it reminds you of some of the blessings you have received in your own life. I hope you consider making your own gratitude list.

Gratitude

- My God. I am grateful to have come to faith, to confess myself as a sinner, to be forgiven and loved by God who sent his only Son to die for me that I may have eternal life. All power, glory, and honor to you, Lord.
- My husband Dan, who really is and always will be my knight in shining armor, who saved me in all the ways one person can save another person by his love and by sharing his faith with me. I am eternally grateful, literally.
- My daughter Emily who has a very kind heart and a beautiful soul. She sometimes articulates wisdom and compassion beyond her years.
- My daughter Sarah, who also has a kind heart and a beautiful soul. Her music blesses this household and my lucky ears.
- My parents who deeply and completely loved me to the best of their ability.
- My in-laws who put God and keeping loving relationships above winning any sort of argument every time.
- My friends: caring, listening, questions, *hugs*, food, flowers, books, cards, e-mails, and so much more.
- Kate: walking this walk with me, a support group of two as we went through treatment together.
- I am grateful for not going through this alone. I am hugely grateful for that.

- My published book to share my ideas to help others.
- My publisher, O Books, who helped me promote my first book, and Ayni Books who have accepted this book!
- My publicist, Ascot Media, who prayed, expressed empathy and kindness and supported me through the entire experience. Thank you, Trish Stevens!
- Coffee dates with girlfriends!
- Overcoming my speaking anxiety to help others.
- Dark, dark chocolate.
- Fresh and dried fruit.
- Greek yogurt and ground flax.
- A fresh avocado.
- Travel to cool places—including Victoria, Vancouver Island, Florida, Mexico, the Caribbean, Hawaii…
- The smell of coffee, and, of course, the caffeine. How happy I was to learn that coffee is very, very high in antioxidants too!
- Music. It soothes, entertains, and educates the soul.
- Hugs from my husband Dan—his smell and feel.
- The expression in Dan's eyes when he looks at me.
- The dogs—their unconditional love, their smell, and their adorable expressions.
- Quiet mornings at home while the girls are still sleeping.
- Leslie Sansone's *Walk Away the Pounds* DVDs.
- Sandi T, my oncology therapist, who radiates an aura of calm and truly has a passion and talent for helping people battle their cancer on all fronts.
- Heidi G, oncology nutritionist, whose willingness to answer questions, enthusiasm about food, and knowledge of nutrition are boundless.
- Mary S, who understands, learns, and helps with the physical therapy and healing process.
- *Everybody Loves Raymond, Cheers, The Wonder Years, The Dick Van Dyke Show, Mad About You, Frasier, 30 Rock, That 70's Show, Mary Tyler Moore…*

What does your gratitude list look like? Could you make it a habit to add an item or two every day? Again, it is about perspective and focus. What are you looking at?

Purpose Tool

After a traumatic life-changing event, has your purpose changed? That may seem like a strange question. It is a personal question, and it depends on where you were going into this and where you are now. You may find it a relief to get back to your normal activities and employment. You may decide or feel like you want to make some changes.

This next list is a bit of a surprise. It reflects effort to find meaning, and yet it looks pretty forward-minded. In fact, it looks kind of like goal setting, which was a concept that is hard to consider when living moment to moment in active cancer treatment.

Barb's Search for Meaning List
(her personal work in progress begun June 28, 2010)

1. Love and serve God.
2. Love and serve my family.
3. Love and serve my friends.
4. Practice compassion.
5. Help get the message of my book out to help others. Live my speaking-writing passion.
6. Find the parts of my life that aren't broken and hang out there.
7. Weave cancer into the fabric of my life. It doesn't change the color or shape of the fabric. It is like a quilt in that it gets a patch, and like a woven textile in that it adds some threads of a new shade and pattern that weren't there before.

8. Create a "new normal" for myself.
9. Choose and support a cancer cause. Cancer awareness, support, and research.
10. Participate in cancer studies if possible. Volunteer to help others behind me on this path.
11. Work on my bucket list.

What is *your* purpose? What do you want? What are your goals? Cancer survivors can't help but be more aware of our own mortality after what we have been through. We, of all people, truly know our days are numbered. We no longer have the luxury/gift/curse of not knowing that our days are numbered. How do you want to spend your days? I am a frugal person and careful with my money, but even I know that ultimately how I spend my time is way more important to me now than how I spend my money.

These thoughts are meant to inspire and not invoke any "shoulds" for you. While engaging in a little self-beating over coffee and conversation with a fellow survivor, she wrote down an important thing for me to tell myself that I would like you to find comfort in too: "I am always doing the best I can!"

Period.

Still a Marathon

Hey, this is still a marathon! Diagnosis happened quite a while ago (though the details may still be vivid as though it was yesterday). Treatment was physically and mentally and emotionally difficult. After active treatment, no one is poking at you as frequently to test or treat anything. It may feel great that active treatment has stopped, and/or it may feel a little like swinging on a trapeze without a safety net!

I repeat: This is still a marathon. Hair may be growing (or already have grown) back. Color may have returned to your face. You may look normal, but on the inside you may be feeling anything *but* normal. Sometimes it's nice to be an attention getter, even if it is by having cancer(!), but it is important to move forward now too.

I had some cancer observations during my journey. I am not sure how this list started. I found keeping the list below helpful. If you decide to have a list like this, it is never too early or late in your cancer journey. Again, the point is to get these thoughts and feelings out of spinning around and around in your head and put down on paper. It can help make them more manageable. It can help you begin to release some of those thoughts and feelings as you move forward.

Cancer Observations (ongoing)

1. I feel very, very, very alone.
2. I feel very, very, very loved.
3. I feel loved just for me, not for what I accomplish.
4. I am very anxious, sad and *scared*, and even angry.
5. I think and hope I am learning to be a more compassionate and caring person.
6. I have prayed more than I have ever prayed before.
7. I have read my Bible more often.
8. It hurt to let other people clean my house.
9. I want my life back.
10. I am not sure what that life "should" look like now.
11. Friends call to check on me. I don't feel worthy. I am deeply grateful.
12. How can I beat this with the required positive attitude, if, by nature, I am more of a glass-is-half-empty sort of a person?
13. Can I give this any meaning? How can I turn this into a

positive? How can I help other people? How can I look further than a few days down the road? Emotions run really, really strong sometimes.

14. Sometimes there are fewer emotions and I am just tired of having cancer.

15. My life didn't go away, but my brain (90%) has moved away from my life.

16. I am working to get my life back piece by piece.

17. This will be *a healthy lifestyle change* that I had started a few months before the diagnosis. Here is the nutritionist's statistic: *A healthy diet and lifestyle can reduce recurrence by 42%!*

18. I am tired of having had breast cancer. Have I mentioned that yet?

19. Sometimes I try the things on the self-help for breast cancer list to the point of exhaustion, and it still doesn't help.

20. Healing from breast cancer is a marathon, not a sprint. I am better at sprints.

21. I am an impatient person. I am an "instant gratification seeker" type of a person. I can learn this skill. I may not be a natural with patience, but I can do better.

You can make your own list. You *can* sort through this stuff moment by moment, day by day, week by week... you get the idea.

Cancer Sometimes Comes Back
(the same cancer—or a completely different cancer)

Life doesn't come with a map.
Sarah Tako

I believe there are some statistics that show that people who have had a first cancer are more likely to get cancer than those who have never had cancer. It could be a recurrence, a new cancer of the same type, or a different kind of cancer than the first cancer. It is information to be aware of but not to dwell on, if you ask me. Again, it seems to come back to the uncertainty that cancer survivors live with daily. It is hard on people to have constant uncertainty. Almost four years out from my breast cancer, I had another unrelated cancer:

February 19, 2014:
I feel like I could have worked on my book today but after being handed the pea-sized lymph node above my right collarbone to worry about for the next 3 weeks (including over a winter vacation), I just don't want to face my cancer book. I was in for a regular check with my vascular doctor who spotted the node. I felt blindsided because I went to that appointment to monitor my lymphedema and I wasn't expecting to hear anything cancer-related. I wasn't expecting to have a new cancer worry handed to me.

I know that not everything is cancer. I know this is probably nothing. I still am tired and frustrated and worried to have this given to me to keep track of and to actively remind me of my cancer. I haven't told anyone but Dan. I don't want to cry wolf all the time, but I feel like I would like the prayers/support too. As for the support, I sort of want to try to manage this worry myself. I will allow myself flexibility in approaching this worry.

March 14, 2014:
After our vacation, I was diagnosed with a melanoma in situ (Stage 0) on my left shoulder. I requested a second lab opinion because of previous conflicting pathology reports on another mole a couple years ago.

March 18, 2014:

I learned the CAT scan of the lymph node and lungs (I was worried about a lingering cough) came back fine, but I was told that I should ask my breast cancer surgeon to check the lymph node out too when I see her in a couple of months. Another lingering thing to manage... Yuck!

March 27, 2014:

The second lab says my melanoma is Stage 1A, not in situ (not Stage 0). The dermatology surgeon will do an outpatient larger excision of the area with deeper and wider margins and there will be a final pathology report. It is a lentigo maligma melanoma that my dermatologist says is "slightly invasive." My dermatologist thinks the confusion between the two lab reports has to do with whether or not each is counting the mole that surrounds the melanoma or not. She and her assistant have been wonderful with promptly returning phone calls and answering my list of questions as it has grown. My doctor also reassures me that my particular melanoma pathology report has an extremely low recurrence and metastasizing rate.

From what I can read, it appears this type of skin cancer may have a fairly high recurrence rate but low chance of spreading. My dermatologist will now see me every 3 months for 2 years for a full body check to monitor me carefully.

I get off the phone in tears and fears. I want to feel safe. The world isn't safe. Life isn't safe. As my therapist says, life is messy. I want guarantees. I want my 100% certainty and perfect test score. The real world doesn't work that way. I feel afraid and not very resilient at all. The anxiety-depression struggles and previous breast cancer experience and the lymph node and the CAT scan that showed on my breast what is "probably" just old scar tissue add to my angst. I have a mammogram next month. I will get through this.

I try to work through my thoughts and feelings: I feel like this is my fault—family history that I was somewhat aware of, lack of sunscreen use, use of tanning beds before vacations. This is sort of like how I used to try to blame myself for my breast cancer—processed foods, alcohol, being overweight. I feel at fault. I share some of my feelings with my friends. I am grateful for their encouragement.

April 21, 2014:

My dermatologist removed six more suspicious things on my skin and addressed my own list of moles. It was very thorough. That felt great! It helped relieve the fear that other things on my skin were lying in wait.

April 25, 2014:

I learn that four of the additional moles removed are normal, and one is moderately atypical and needs to be watched for regrowth, and one is severely atypical, but not cancer, and I need to go back to have surgically wider margins for that one. I am relieved but still feeling anxious about my upcoming 4-year mammogram and worried about the lymph node up above my right collarbone. I am weary of the waiting and watching.

Finding out I had a melanoma, often called the deadliest form of skin cancer, was both the same as and different from hearing I had breast cancer the first time.

Time froze a little when I got the call. I remember thinking it wasn't good that the doctor was calling with the results herself rather than hearing from her assistant. I was better at asking some of the medical questions because I had previous experience. I was scared. I felt singled out. I felt guilty, especially for using a tanning bed a little before our vacation this winter, especially because I, of all people, should know better. I was already struggling with some anxiety-depression and then I was thrown this curve ball too. Hearing the new worries and eventual diagnosis aggravated the anxiety-depression feelings and the PTSD. I struggled with the wait—to get a second lab's opinion on the sample (my request) and the scheduled wait for the appointment to have the more extensive excision surgery to be sure that all of it got removed with clear margins.

My upper left arm meligma melanoma was excised several weeks ago. I was told to wear sunscreen and sent home with a catalog of sun-blocking clothing that reminded me of the wig catalog I was given with chemo for breast cancer. On one hand, it wasn't my first rodeo and I had moments I felt okay. On the other hand, it was a second cancer! Like a second baby, no one around me reacted much, but *I* was very upset! I didn't want or necessarily need a lot of attention, but I felt like I needed the people around me to be able to listen a little and give me time to process the second cancer. I needed time and support to learn how to wrap my head around this second cancer. Life continued to go on anyway and it didn't seem to slow down for much of that.

I was gentler with myself this time. I would cry when I needed to cry. I tried to focus on the tactile at times: I would curl up under a soft blanket and focus on the feel and comfort from it, as well as appreciating my two dogs who often joined in on either side to protect me. I tried to focus on the senses. I would close my eyes and categorize the sounds. I would listen to a guided imagery exercise. I tried to stay in the moment. In short, I used my survival tools and they helped. They didn't solve every feeling, but they helped. I also went back on the anxiety medication that I had weaned off of toward the end of last year. I may try to reduce the dosage at some point, but I don't think I will try to wean completely off again.

If I had any advice to share from this experience it would be: Be vigilant about your health and doctor appointments and also be vigilant about your emotions and mental health if a second cancer or other health or life crisis comes. Remember and use the emotional tools in your backpack that you have learned. Above all, be gentle with yourself.

Fear of Recurrence

August 20, 2014:

Has my breast cancer or melanoma spread? I went to my generalist doctor in fear and this time left in hope. I had found a lump on the top of my hand and rather than it being anything dire, it turned out to be nothing more than a common ganglion cyst. He was very kind and reassuring. He understood where I was emotionally because of my past experiences. Breathe. Celebrate the relief.

I know it won't be the last time I run to the doctor with a cancer recurrence worry in my mind *and* I get back to my life as soon as I can. You will learn this skill too. You will get there.

I try to remember that not everything that happens to my body as I age is cancer. I will get colds, flu, and struggle with arthritis and more. I remind myself that is it "normal" to be afraid of recurrence after having had cancer. The cancer fears can return so quickly when any health issue comes up or a worry enters my mind. Once again, it is important to remember that the fear is a normal feeling for an abnormal situation. The loss of certainty is real and I can work through it *and* I can live my life. When worries arise, see a doctor. Resolve the worries and don't let them nag at you. More research and resources are coming out every day to help survivors. We are not alone.

Conclusions and Celebrations

What do we live for, if it is not to make life less difficult for each other?
George Eliot

Congratulations! You can do this. You are doing this. You have done this. You may be in a hurry to move forward or back to "normal" life, but it would be a shame not to give yourself the credit for getting through this that you earned and deserve. You have faced down the Boogie Man named Cancer and moved forward past him. That is worth celebrating.

Writing to Others Tool

Continue to journal—it may help you realize the progress you are making in creating your "new normal." Writing to friends and family who supported you on your journey is also a tool. Writing to those who supported you on this journey may help you to practice gratitude, to wrap things up, and to move forward.

Here is an e-mail I sent to my kind, concerned supporters a couple months after breast cancer treatments ended:

I wanted to write a New Year's thank-you note to you. I could not have gotten through the past eight months without God and you! To call it a challenging journey would be a trite understatement. I honestly hope, as I try to create a "new normal" from here forward, that I won't forget some of the important lessons I learned, and I definitely want to be in the lives of the really awesome people I met and/or came into closer or more frequent contact with because of the breast cancer. I am so grateful to you.

Speaking of gratitude, I find myself grateful for many small normal things that have returned or are in the process of returning. Think of Julie Andrews singing, "These are a few of my favorite things" — When the hair grows, when the food tastes, when the normal bra is back... Okay, enough already.

I went into this experience as a selfish, hectic, and worried person. I hope I am leaving this portion of my life journey as a more caring, rational, and calm person — with adjusted priorities, my face turned more toward God, and a deeper gratitude for what is important in this life. I hope I will be able to move forward and at the same time continue to process and remember what I learned from this experience. I will say this, there is *good* that came of this experience. No doubt about it. You are part of that goodness.

Above all, *you* are important to me. Thank *you* for being there for me.

Here are two timely quotes that I recently found:

"Scar tissue is stronger than regular tissue.
Realize the strength, move on."
—Henry Rollins

"The great lesson ... is that the sacred is in the ordinary; that it is to be found in one's daily life, in one's neighbors, friends, and family, in one's backyard."
—Abraham Maslow

I wish you a joyous and peaceful New Year, and once again, I send you my deepest thanks.

Love, Barb

Writing one or several thank-you notes or letters may be another coping tool for you. It gives you a chance to reflect and gain perspective. It helps you foster an attitude of gratitude. It helps you see and realize that you are moving forward and recognizes all that you have accomplished.

Waiting for the Cancer *Not* to Come Back

Cancer does not consume every waking moment and every thought of every day for me anymore.

Over four years out from breast cancer diagnosis and definitely two years out from lumpectomy, chemo and radiation, and just a few months past the melanoma, how do I feel? Better? Calmer? Grateful? Yes, yes, and definitely yes. Am I "back to normal"? I don't think so. There is no old normal. The doctors won't say, "Cured." Instead, they tell me, "Heal, get back to your life, and we will wait and watch."

I don't like the "wait and watch" part. I get to move on but I don't get to be done. Sometimes I worry if I have a cough or a pain. Sometimes I don't worry. Other times, I worry later that maybe I should have worried, and there I am around the circle and back, not to the beginning, but back to "wait and watch." I am grateful that I am still here. I appreciate the people around me more. I enjoy the little things more. I resent the time, energy and peace that waiting and watching sometimes steal.

Limbo isn't a comfortable place, maybe because we don't have a lot of practice living in limbo in our instant-gratification, "ships in the next 24 hours" type of society. Living with uncertainty can be hard on people. Maybe some of us have had more experience with limbo than others. Dealing with being in limbo just isn't easy for many of us.

Is there a trick to handling it? There are many ways to handle it. I think it comes down to processing, time, and a matter of focus. Processing means not stuffing the feelings of worry when they pop up. It means we get to work through our feelings. The feelings, again, are normal for an abnormal situation. The feelings, and the scary thoughts that come with them, get to say their piece and have their time for me to work through them. The other side of the same coin, though, is for me to decide how much of my time those thoughts and feelings get, and that brings me to focus.

Some women choose to focus on and identify more with their breast cancer experience. They may have met fellow survivor friends and they may choose to actively support others with cancer or efforts to cure cancer. They may choose to help others not as far along on their cancer journey. They may stay in a support group for months or years after their treatment. Other women get pulled back into the demands of the life they had before cancer. The cancer isn't forgotten. It is just that they choose to place more focus on the things they did before the cancer or the things that currently demand their attention because the rest of the world wasn't standing still while they went through their cancer treatment.

Those two directions aren't really an "either/or" situation. As individuals, we each get to choose how much of our focus we place on cancer in general, on our personal wait in limbo, on our life after cancer, and on how much being a cancer survivor defines us. I think of my focus sort of like a stage spotlight. I can widen and narrow the spotlight, and I can choose where I point it, and I can move it around.

Sometimes my spotlight shines on my anger and resentment. Sometimes it swings over to my fear or uncertainty. Other times, the spotlight highlights humor or wisdom. It also shines on gratitude and peace. Where are you pointing your spotlight right now? You can choose. You can do this. You *are* doing this.

Bucket List Tool

Write down your bucket list items and work on checking them off! You can even write down the ones you have already done and check them off too. Live your life right now! You can make and achieve your plans. You can get out there and do this!

Edited from the Internet (source unknown):
Subject: Shoulda, woulda, coulda
Too many people put off something that brings them joy just because they haven't thought about it, don't have it on their schedule, didn't know it was coming or are too rigid to depart from their routine.

I got to thinking one day about all those people on the *Titanic* who passed up dessert at dinner that fateful night in an effort to cut back. From then on, I've tried to be a little more flexible. How many women out there will eat at home because their husband didn't suggest going out to dinner until after something had been thawed? Does the word "refrigeration" mean nothing to you?

How often have your kids dropped in to talk and sat in silence while you watched *Jeopardy* on television? I cannot count the times I called my sister and said, "How about going to lunch in a half hour?" She would gas up and stammer, "I can't. I have clothes on the line. My hair is dirty. I wish I had known yesterday. I had a late breakfast. It looks like rain." And my personal favorite: "It's Monday." She died a few days ago. We never did have lunch together. Because we cram so much into our lives, we tend to schedule our headaches. We live on a sparse diet of promises we make to ourselves when all the conditions are perfect! We'll go back and visit the grandparents when we get Steve toilet-trained. We'll entertain when we replace the living-room carpet. We'll go on a second honeymoon when we get two more kids out of college. Life has a way of accelerating as we get older. The days get shorter, and the list of promises to ourselves gets longer. One morning, we awaken, and all we have to show for our lives is a litany of "I'm going to," "I plan on," and "Someday, when things are settled down a bit."

When anyone calls my "seize the moment" friend, she is open to adventure and available for trips. She keeps an open mind on new ideas. Her enthusiasm for life is contagious. You talk with her for five minutes, and you're ready to trade your bad feet for a pair of rollerblades and skip an elevator for a bungee cord.

My lips have not touched ice cream in 10 years. I love ice cream. It's just that I might as well apply it directly to my stomach with a spatula and eliminate the digestive process. The other day, I stopped the car and bought a triple-decker. If my car had hit an iceberg on the way home, I would have died happy.

Now... go on and have a nice day. Do something you *want* to... not something on your *should do* list. If you were going to die soon and had only one phone call you could make, who would you call and what would you say? And why are you waiting? I had a friend from high school that I was always going to call and never did. The other day her name was in the obituaries so we never had that chat.

> Have you ever watched kids playing on a merry-go-round
> or listened to the rain lapping on the ground?
> Ever followed a butterfly's erratic flight
> or gazed at the sun into the fading night?
> Do you run through each day on the fly?
> When you ask, "How are you?" do you hear the reply?
> When the day is done, do you lie in your bed
> with the next hundred chores running through your head?
> Ever told your child, "We'll do it tomorrow,"
> and in your haste, not see his sorrow?

Ever lost touch? Let a good friendship die?
Just call to say "Hi"?
When you worry and hurry through your day,
it is like an unopened gift... thrown away...
Life is not a race. Take it slower.
Hear the music before the song is over.
Tell your friends:
"Life may not be the party we hoped for...
but while we are here we might as well dance!"

Today my hair isn't falling out
by Barbara Tako

Today my hair isn't falling out.
It is partly cloudy.

Today chemo isn't coursing through my body.
I catch myself humming along with the song on the radio.

Today I am not having post-surgery pain.
I can run errands.

Today I am not thinking about cancer every minute of every
hour of every day.
I can buy groceries for tomorrow.

Today, right now, this moment is just for me to be.
Thank you, God, for right now.

Afterword

At this moment, I am over four years out from the breast cancer diagnosis and a few months out from the melanoma. Do I worry about the cancers coming back? Yes. Does it occupy every second of my thoughts? No. Life has brought other challenges since the cancers—experiencing what it is like to be an empty nester, moving my parents closer to me as they aged and needed an assisted-living residence near me, the death of my dad, helping my mom through her grief and her own recently discovered breast cancer and advanced glaucoma, and more.

In short, life, during and after getting through cancer, just keeps on happening. I try to work through all of it as best I can. Sometimes there are good days. Sometimes there are bad days. I fare best when I can take a breath, be loose, and go with the flow. In that breath, that momentary pause to breathe and listen, I can see infinite possibilities in how I choose to react to life's bumps and glitches. Sometimes I can make better choices than I would have in the past. I like to think that working through the cancers has helped to teach me that. Some moments, it is easier to practice that philosophy than others.

I hope the journal entries shared in this book help you to understand and feel that you are not alone on your journey. I hope the tools in this book help you cope with your cancer and your life. If there are items in this book that rub you the wrong way, I hope you understand that is entirely my fault and problem, not yours. Please take the good and freely discard the rest.

I wish you longer and longer moments of peace and joy and wisdom as you continue through your journey and your life.

Blessings,

Barb

Share your cancer journey and inspiration

Send Barbara Tako an email:
  barbaratako@gmail.com

See Barbara's website:
  www.cancersurvivorshipcopingtools.com

Or write to Barbara Tako at:
  Barbara Tako
  Ayni Books
  The Bothy
  Deershot Lodge
  Park Lane
  Ropley
  Hants
  SO24 0BE
  United Kingdom

Bibliography and Further Reading

Callister, Sharon. *On Wings of the Dawn: A devotional book for women experiencing breast cancer and their supporters* (Beaver's Pond Press Inc., 2003).

Chodron, Pema. *When Things Fall Apart: Heart advice for difficult times* (Shambhala, 1997).

Delinsky, Barbara. *Uplift: Secrets from the sisterhood of breast cancer survivors* (Washington Square Press, 2006).

Emmons, Henry, MD. *The Chemistry of Calm: Settle your mind – Reclaim healthy emotions – Stop worrying and start fully living!* (Touchstone, a division of Simon & Schuster, Inc., 2010).

GRQ Inc. *Moments of Peace for a Woman's Heart: Reflections of God's gifts of love, hope, and comfort* (Bethany House Publishers, 2008).

LeShan, Lawrence. *How to Meditate: A guide to self-discovery* (Little, Brown and Company, 1999).

Rinpoche, Yongey Mingyur with Eric Swanson. *The Joy of Living: Unlocking the secret and science of happiness* (Three Rivers Press, 2007).

Tako, Barbara. *Clutter Clearing Choices: Clear clutter, organize your home, and reclaim your life* (O Books, 2010).

Walker, Laura Jensen. *Thanks for the Mammogram!* (Fleming H. Revell, a division of Baker Book House Company, 2000).

Website Resources

(Disclaimer: The resources mentioned below were personally helpful to me during treatment. I was a cancer patient, not a resource expert. The resources that you choose may be different. As always: Choose carefully. Ask people you trust. Move on to a different source if something bothers you.)

ACS—American Cancer Society at http://www.cancer.org/ has resources about cancer, health, treatment, research, and volunteering.

AICR at http://www.aicr.org/ "funds cutting-edge research and gives people practical tools and information to help them prevent and survive cancer."

NCI—National Cancer Institute at http://www.cancer.gov/ is "the federal government's principal agency for cancer research and training." They also provide health information regarding the "causes, diagnosis, prevention, and treatment of cancer, rehabilitation from cancer, and the continuing care of cancer patients and the families of cancer patients."

Dr. Susan Love Research Foundation at http://www.dslrf.org/ "provides comprehensive information about breast cancer, menopause, women's health, and ductal lavage…"

Breastcancer.org at http://www.breastcancer.org provides information about breast cancer and breast health as well as an online support community.

LiveStrong.org at http://www.livestrong.org is an organization that works to help improve the lives of people affected by cancer.

Proverbs 31 Ministries at http://www.proverbs31.org is a non-denominational, non-profit Christian ministry that offers free devotions, a daily radio message, speaking events, conferences, resources and more.

Healthjourneys.com at http://www.healthjourneys.com offers guided imagery and other mind–body resources.

EWG at http://www.ewg.org is an environmental health research and advocacy organization that offers consumer resources and information.

SparkPeople.com at http://www.sparkpeople.com helps people lose weight and make healthy lifestyle choices.

The Ripples Project at http://www.theripplesproject.org is a resource of inspirational quotes that offers a weekly newsletter and online community.

AYNI
BOOKS

"Ayni" is a Quechua word meaning "reciprocity" – sharing, giving and receiving – whatever you give out comes back to you. To be in Ayni is to be in balance, harmony and right relationship with oneself and nature, of which we are all an intrinsic part. Complementary and Alternative approaches to health and well-being essentially follow a holistic model, within which one is given support and encouragement to move towards a state of balance, true health and wholeness, ultimately leading to the awareness of one's unique place in the Universal jigsaw of life – Ayni, in fact.